PROMPT

PRactical Obstetric
Multi-Professional Training

Trainer's Manual

Third Edition

Edited by

Cathy Winter, Joanna Crofts, Timothy Draycott
and Neil Muchatuta

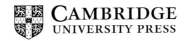

CAMBRIDGE
UNIVERSITY PRESS

CAMBRIDGE
UNIVERSITY PRESS

University Printing House, Cambridge CB2 8BS, United Kingdom

One Liberty Plaza, 20th Floor, New York, NY 10006, USA

477 Williamstown Road, Port Melbourne, VIC 3207, Australia

314–321, 3rd Floor, Plot 3, Splendor Forum, Jasola District Centre, New Delhi – 110025, India

79 Anson Road, #06–04/06, Singapore 079906

Cambridge University Press is part of the University of Cambridge.

It furthers the University's mission by disseminating knowledge in the pursuit of education, learning, and research at the highest international levels of excellence.

www.cambridge.org
Information on this title: www.cambridge.org/9781108433754
DOI: 10.1017/9781108380799

Registered Charity in England and Wales No. 1140557
Registered Company No. 7506593
Registered Office: Stone King LLP, 13 Queen Square, Bath, BA1 2HJ
www.promptmaternity.org

PROMPT Training Permissions and Licences
Units or institutions paying for a multi-professional team to attend an authorised PROMPT Train the Trainers (T3) day are only permitted to run PROMPT multi-professional obstetric emergencies training courses, using PROMPT course materials, within their own unit or institution.

Any PROMPT training conducted outside the unit or institution that has permission (see above) requires a licence from the PROMPT Maternity Foundation (PMF), e.g. a professional organisation or body wishing to roll out PROMPT training within a region or country, or a unit wishing to run PROMPT training at other hospitals outside of their own hospital group.

PMF is happy to discuss licensing arrangements or answer any questions relating to training permissions at any time. Please contact info@promptmaternity.org giving details of the training that is proposed.

Any training tools within this manual are based on national guidance where available, but the PROMPT Maternity Foundation is not a national body. Therefore, we would advise that to use these tools locally, they should be approved by your governance structures after adapting for local use.

First edition published by the Royal College of Obstetricians and Gynaecologists 2008
Second edition published 2012
Third edition published by Cambridge University Press 2018
Reprinted 2020

Printed in the United Kingdom by Clays, St Ives plc

A catalogue record for this publication is available from the British Library.

Library of Congress Cataloging-in-Publication Data
Names: Winter, Cathy (Midwife), editor. | Crofts, Jo (Joanna), editor. |
    Laxton, Chris (Christina), editor. | Barnfield, Sonia, editor. | Draycott,
    Timothy J., editor. | PROMPT Maternity Foundation, sponsoring body.
Title: PROMPT. Trainer's manual / edited by Cathy Winter, Jo Crofts, Chris
    Laxton, Sonia Barnfield and Tim Draycott.
Other titles: Trainer's manual | PRactical Obstetric Multi-Professional
    Training. Trainer's manual | Complemented by (expression): PROMPT course
    manual. Third edition.
Description: Third edition. | Cambridge, United Kingdom ; New York, NY :
    University Printing House, 2017. | Includes bibliographical references.
Identifiers: LCCN 2017046630 | ISBN 9781108433754 (paperback)
Subjects: | MESH: Obstetric Labor Complications | Teaching Materials |
    Obstetrics – education | Emergencies | Teaching
Classification: LCC RG571 | NLM WQ 18.2 | DDC 618.2–dc23
LC record available at https://lccn.loc.gov/2017046630

ISBN 978-1-108-43375-4 Paperback

Contents

Contents

Editorial team and contributors

PROMPT Editorial Team

Joanna Crofts	Consultant Obstetrician, Bristol
Timothy Draycott	Consultant Obstetrician, Bristol
Neil Muchatuta	Consultant Anaesthetist, Bristol
Cathy Winter	Senior Research Midwife, Bristol

Contributors

Ms Mary Alvarez	Senior Research Midwife, Bristol
Lt-Col Tracy-Louise Appleyard	Consultant Obstetrician and Gynaecologist, Bristol/RAMC
Dr Sonia Barnfield	Consultant Obstetrician, Bristol
Ms Andrea Blotkamp	Clinical Fellow in Midwifery, RCOG
Dr Christy Burden	NIHR Academic Clinical Lecturer, University of Bristol
Dr Yealin Chung	Academic Research Fellow, Bristol
Dr Kate Collins	PMF Research Fellow, Bristol
Dr Katie Cornthwaite	NIHR Academic Clinical Fellow, Bristol
Dr Joanna Crofts	Consultant Obstetrician, Bristol
Mr Max Crofts	PMF Volunteer, Bath
Dr Ishita Das	Specialty Trainee in Obstetrics and Gynaecology, Bristol

Dr Fiona Donald	Consultant Anaesthetist, Bristol
Professor Timothy Draycott	Consultant Obstetrician, Bristol
Dr Sian Edwards	Specialty Trainee in Obstetrics and Gynaecology, Gloucester
Dr Islam Gamaleldin	NIHR Academic Clinical Lecturer, University of Bristol
Dr Kiren Ghag	PMF Research Fellow, Bristol
Ms Susan Hughes	Senior Midwife, Bristol
Dr Judith Hyde	Consultant Obstetrician, Bristol
Mr Mark James	Consultant Obstetrician and Gynaecologist, Gloucester
Ms Sharon Jordan	Senior Midwife, Bristol
Dr Christina Laxton	Consultant Anaesthetist, Bristol
Dr Erik Lenguerrand	Medical Statistician, University of Bristol
Ms Mary Lynch	Senior Midwife, Bristol
Ms Lisa Marshall	PMF Midwife Project Manager, Bristol
Dr Neil Muchatuta	Consultant Anaesthetist, Bristol
Dr Helen van der Nelson	Specialty Trainee in Obstetrics and Gynaecology, Gloucester
Dr Stephen O'Brien	PMF Research Fellow, Bristol
Dr Kate O'Connor	Consultant Anaesthetist, Bristol
Dr David Odd	Consultant Neonatologist, Bristol
Ms Beverley Osborne	Senior Midwife, Bristol
Dr Mark Scrutton	Consultant Anaesthetist, Bristol
Ms Debbie Senior	Practice Development Midwife, Bristol
Dr Dimitrios Siassakos	Clinical Lecturer in Obstetrics, University of Bristol
Dr Thabani Sibanda	Consultant Obstetrician, New Zealand
Dr Rebecca Simms	Consultant Obstetrician, Bristol

Ms Debbie Sirett	PMF Support Manager, Bristol
Ms Angie Sledge	Senior Midwife, Bristol
Ms Ellie Sonmezer	Senior Midwife, Gloucester
Dr Maria Tsakmakis	Consultant Neonatologist, Bristol
Dr Tim Walker	Specialty Doctor in Anaesthetics, Bristol
Dr Nicky Weale	Consultant Anaesthetist, Bristol
Ms Heather Wilcox	Senior Midwife, Bristol
Mr Nigel Williams	PMF Voluntary Legal Advisor, Wales
Ms Cathy Winter	PMF Senior Research Midwife, Bristol
Ms Meg Winter	PMF Volunteer, Bristol
Ms Stephanie Withers	Practice Development Midwife, Bristol
Ms Elaine Yard	Senior Midwife, Bristol
Dr Christopher Yau	PMF Research Fellow, Bristol

Acknowledgements

The PROMPT Maternity Foundation (PMF) is a registered charity in England and Wales (Charity No. 1140557). The aim of the charity is to improve awareness and facilitate the distribution of effective, multi-professional, obstetric emergencies training as widely as possible to areas of the world requesting access to an economical and sustainable training model.

Over the past 5 years, there has been increasing evidence that the PROMPT method of training for maternity emergencies is having a significant impact, not only in the UK but internationally. In 2016, PROMPT training was recognised in the NHS England National Maternity Review, *Better Births*.

The growth and increasing recognition of PROMPT training is underpinned by robust research, collecting further evidence to support the improvements in outcomes seen in some maternity units in the UK and across the globe. PMF research projects are funded through fundraising, corporate partnerships and research grants from both UK and international bodies.

Internationally, PROMPT is now being taught in the USA, Australia, New Zealand, Zimbabwe, Laos, Abu Dhabi and UAE, Singapore, Hong Kong, Philippines, Switzerland, France, Germany, Spain and the West Indies.

This is the third edition of the PROMPT *Trainer's Manual,* and it has been developed and produced with the help of:

- Maternity staff of North Bristol NHS Trust
- The PROMPT Maternity Foundation trustees, members, researchers and facilitators
- Maternity teams that attended the PROMPT 3 Pilot T3 training from the South West Obstetric Network, Bolton NHS Trust and St Thomas' Hospital, London
- Limbs & Things
- Laerdal Medical
- The Health Foundation

The final production of the third edition of the PROMPT course would not have been possible without the invaluable commitment and support of:

- The Louise Stratton Memorial Fund – whose fundraising projects enabled the very first PROMPT training package to be produced.

- All the volunteers and supporters who have held fundraising activities on behalf of the PROMPT Maternity Foundation.

- Christopher Eskell – Chief Executive Officer (CEO) of the PROMPT Maternity Foundation (2011–2016), who sadly died in October 2016 after a short illness. He was the CEO of PMF for 5 years, and thanks to his skill and dedication, PROMPT has grown from a small Bristol project into an international gold standard for training. Thank you to Christopher for his contribution to creating our charity, and for his meticulous work underpinning all of our successes.

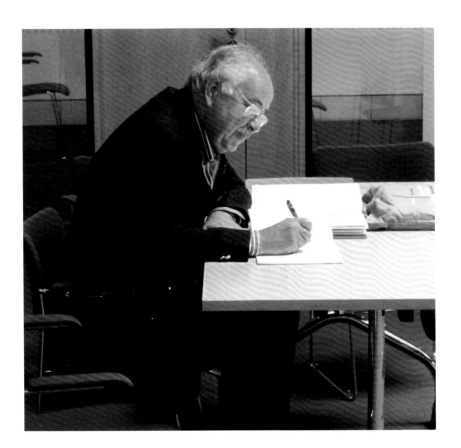

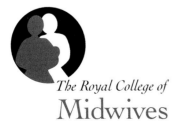

The Royal College of
Midwives

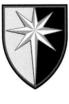

Royal College of
Obstetricians and Gynaecologists

Bringing to life the best in women's health care

Obstetric
Anaesthetists'
Association

Abbreviations and terms

AAGBI	Association of Anaesthetists of Great Britain and Ireland
ABC	airway, breathing, circulation
ABCDE	airway, breathing, circulation, disability, exposure
AED	automated external defibrillator
ALS	advanced life support
APH	antepartum haemorrhage
ARM	artificial rupture of membranes
BLS	basic life support
BMI	body mass index
BP	blood pressure
bpm	beats per minute
CICO	can't intubate can't oxygenate
CMACE	Centre for Maternal and Child Enquiries
CPR	cardiopulmonary resuscitation
CRP	C-reactive protein
CS	caesarean section
CTG	cardiotocograph
DAS	Difficult Airway Society
EBL	estimated blood loss
ECG	electrocardiogram
EFM	electronic fetal monitoring
EUA	examination under anaesthetic
FBC	full blood count
FBS	fetal blood sample
FFP	fresh frozen plasma
FHR	fetal heart rate
FIGO	International Federation of Gynaecology and Obstetrics
FiO_2	fraction of inspired oxygen
GA	general anaesthesia

GI	gastrointestinal
GP	general practitioner
GTN	glyceryl trinitrate
HCA	healthcare assistant
IA	intermittent auscultation
ICU	intensive care unit
IM	intramuscular
IO	intraosseous
IPPV	intermittent positive pressure ventilation
IV	intravenous
LA	local anaesthetic
LFT	liver function test
LMA	laryngeal mask airway
LMWH	low-molecular-weight heparin
MBRRACE-UK	Mothers and Babies: Reducing Risk through Audits and Confidential Enquiries across the UK
MCA	maternity care assistant
MOEWS	Modified Obstetric Early Warning Score
NHS	National Health Service
NIBP	non-invasive blood pressure
NICE	National Institute for Health and Care Excellence
NLS	newborn life support
NSAID	non-steroidal anti-inflammatory drug
OA	occipito-anterior
OAA	Obstetric Anaesthetists' Association
ODP	operating department practitioner
OVB	operative vaginal birth
PEA	pulseless electrical activity
PPH	postpartum haemorrhage
RBC	red blood cells
RCOG	Royal College of Obstetricians and Gynaecologists
RR	respiratory rate
SBAR	situation, background, assessment and recommendation/response

SpO$_2$	peripheral capillary oxygen saturation
T3	Train the Trainers
TXA	tranexamic acid
U&E	urea and electrolytes
UKOSS	United Kingdom Obstetric Surveillance System
VE	vaginal examination
VF	ventricular fibrillation
VT	ventricular tachycardia
VTE	venous thromboembolism
WOMAN trial	World Maternal Antifibrinolytic trial

Introduction

We hope this third edition of the PROMPT *Trainer's Manual* provides the guidance and materials you need to facilitate the implementation of local PROMPT courses in your own unit or institution. The manual is part of the PROMPT course and is an adjunct to the PROMPT Train the Trainers (T3) programme.

The *Trainer's Manual* is divided into sections and provides specific drill scenarios, scripts, equipment lists and debriefing checklists for all the maternity emergencies described in the third edition of the PROMPT *Course Manual*. It has been revised and updated, and we have added a new section on maternal critical care (Section 13) to reflect the increasing challenges in maternity care.

As part of the PROMPT 'course in a box' you will be able to download PowerPoint presentations, treatment algorithms and documentation tools, and clinical and teamwork checklists to accompany the simulated scenarios/drills, as well as course evaluation sheets and certificates. This download icon is used throughout the manual to identify when a presentation, video clip or training tool can be downloaded for use on your local training courses.

The PROMPT team has over 15 years of experience of local multi-professional obstetric emergencies training. We have endeavoured to share this experience as widely as possible throughout the PROMPT manuals, presentations, tools and cognitive aids in order to facilitate the provision of effective multi-professional maternity training locally.

Most importantly, we have continued to investigate the effectiveness of local PROMPT training, particularly concerning improvements in outcomes for mothers and babies. Based on this evidence, we have included an additional section on local PROMPT implementation (Section 3).

Section 1
Course preparation and administration

Introduction

It is important that all trainers are well prepared and familiar with the contents of the third edition of the PROMPT 'course in a box' prior to running their local PROMPT courses. Therefore, having attended the Train the Trainers (T3) programme, it is a good idea for the local multi-professional training team to meet together in their own institution to review all of the training materials and the downloadable supporting information, in preparation for planning their local courses.

Planning meeting

The local training team should hold a planning meeting to decide course dates, finalise the course programme and organise the venue. They should allocate individual modules to specific trainers, who can then assemble a multi-professional team of staff to organise the required equipment and allocate at least one midwife and one doctor from their team to run the station on each of the training days. It is often useful to practise the scenarios before the first course date, in order to address any problems that may arise and make any necessary local adaptations.

Booking the dates and the venue, and assembling any equipment required well in advance, will minimise problems on the training day itself.

Course programmes

We have included in the downloadable training materials several examples of course programmes, with a selection of different options for PROMPT workshops and scenarios (see Appendix 1). However, we encourage you to tailor the programme to meet the specific requirements of your unit and your local training needs analysis. **It is also important to remember that your local maternity clinical teams are responsible for the content and governance of your local PROMPT courses.**

Course programmes 1 and 2

Programmes 1 and 2 would be best suited for smaller groups of participants: we suggest four multi-professional teams with six participants in each team. The lecture/drill/lecture format would also require the lecture room to be close to the labour ward, as there are several moves to and from the clinical area throughout the day, which would be time-consuming if the distances were too great.

Course programmes 3 and 4

Programmes 3 and 4 are best suited for larger groups: we suggest six multi-professional teams with six to eight participants in each team. All the lectures and workshops are held in one venue in the morning and then all the teams relocate to the clinical area in the afternoon for the drills and hands-on sessions. This means that the room used for lectures in the morning can be further from the clinical area if necessary.

It can be difficult to fit all the subjects and sessions that you need to cover into one training day, so it may be worth considering having some poster stations where staff can read information during their coffee and lunch breaks. This can be another useful way of ensuring staff are updated with local guidance and documentation etc., and A4-sized versions of the posters can also be included in the local pre-reading workbooks (Figures 1.1 and 1.2).

Location of practical workshops and drills

Where possible, the emergency drills should be undertaken in the actual labour ward rooms (in the birth centre, on the labour ward or in the maternal critical care rooms, depending on the scenarios) or other appropriate clinical areas, such as obstetric theatres for the anaesthetic emergencies. The highest environmental fidelity for training venues is the local clinical area. A suitable seminar room (near the labour ward if possible) can also be identified for lectures. However, the availability of clinical rooms for training sessions can be problematic to organise, as there may not be enough empty rooms on the day; the course may also be perceived as an added inconvenience to clinical staff on an already very busy labour

CALL FOR HELP – including midwife coordinator, experienced obstetrician and neonatal team.
Ensure continuous electronic fetal monitoring. Encourage woman into semi-recumbent/all-fours position*
(*Inform mother that recourse to semi-recumbent position may be necessary depending on accoucheur experience and preference of mother)

'HANDS OFF' THE BREECH AS MUCH AS POSSIBLE

Await visualisation of breech at perineum before encouraging active pushing.

Allow 'HANDS-OFF' birth of buttocks and legs. If legs require assistance apply gentle pressure behind baby's knees.

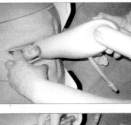
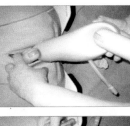
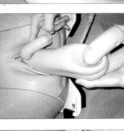
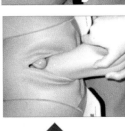

Allow 'HANDS-OFF' birth of body and arms. If arms require assistance perform Lovsett's manoeuvre, ONLY hold baby over hip bones (pelvic girdle), turning baby's body towards the left and right and keeping the back uppermost to release arms.

Remember to document all actions and manoeuvres and fully explain the events to the parents.

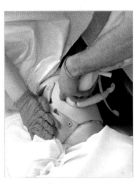

Birth of the baby's head may also be facilitated by an assistant applying suprapubic pressure to encourage flexion of the baby's head.

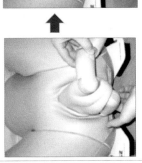
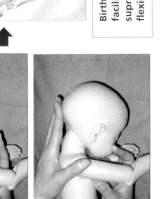
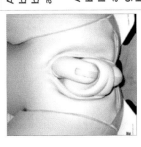

Allow 'HANDS-OFF' birth of shoulders and neck. When the nape of neck is visible, flex baby's head by placing fingers of one hand on the baby's shoulders and back of head, and the 1st and 3rd fingers of the other hand on the baby's cheek bones to aid flexion of the head (Mauriceau–Smellie–Veit manoeuvre).

Figure 1.1 Example of a poster presentation for vaginal breech birth

ward. With this in mind, trainers will need to liaise with the labour ward coordinator regarding rooms that can be used on the day, and if necessary they may need to adapt their scenarios to other training environments.

The benefits of training in the actual clinical environment where real emergencies occur, and with the staff that may actually be called to manage the situation, cannot be overstated. Local training not only enables local protocols and procedures to be tested and, if necessary, revised, but also gives staff a sense of ownership. Often, as a result of participating in drills, staff may suggest simple changes to the location of emergency equipment or system improvements to streamline processes. Drills can also provide very valuable opportunities to pilot and implement new observation charts, documentation pro formas and revised guidelines with frontline staff.

Listed below are actions that we have taken in our maternity unit to maximise opportunities to train in labour ward rooms and other clinical areas:

- Set the training dates well in advance.
- Limit the number of elective caesarean sections scheduled for the day of the training, so that anaesthetic and midwifery faculty have more chance of being free to teach in the afternoon.
- Identify rooms to be used on the actual day of the training. A timetable of room allocations can then be given to each team leader at lunchtime.

> **It is far better to adapt the course programme and continue with whatever facilities and trainers you have for that day, than to cancel the training day altogether.**

If the labour ward is too busy to accommodate the drills then be flexible and use rooms in the antenatal clinic or on the postnatal wards. You could even set up mock labour rooms in offices or seminar rooms, using photographs of labour ward emergency buzzers and other equipment so that staff can still become familiar with the appearance of their own equipment (see Appendix 3).

Course administration

It is a good idea to appoint one or more course coordinators who will be responsible for the administration of the courses. For example, the practice development midwife and the labour ward lead obstetrician or anaesthetist may take on this role together. Contacting the faculty 2–3 weeks in advance of the course date to confirm their availability is vital to ensuring that all drill stations are adequately manned on the day.

Ideally, annual attendance on the PROMPT course should be mandatory for all maternity staff: midwives, MCAs and HCAs, obstetricians (of all levels), anaesthetists, and theatre staff. The aim is for 100% attendance. The dates can be advertised at the start of the year so that staff can book their place well in advance and also request not to be rostered for clinical work that day.

It is advisable to set up an attendance database that can be checked periodically so that non-attenders can be contacted and advised to attend on the next available date. Repeat non-attenders may be given a date to attend by their line manager/clinical supervisor. Attendance can also be monitored via midwifery annual supervisory reviews and medical staff appraisals.

Course manuals, local pre-reading booklet and equipment

The PROMPT *Course Manual*, and any local pre-reading booklets, should ideally be available for participants 1 or 2 weeks before their course date, so that they have time to read the material and prepare for the day. The local pre-reading booklet can be particularly useful for disseminating local information, new charts, guidelines, the monthly dashboard of local outcomes and photos identifying the location of specific equipment etc. (Figure 1.2).

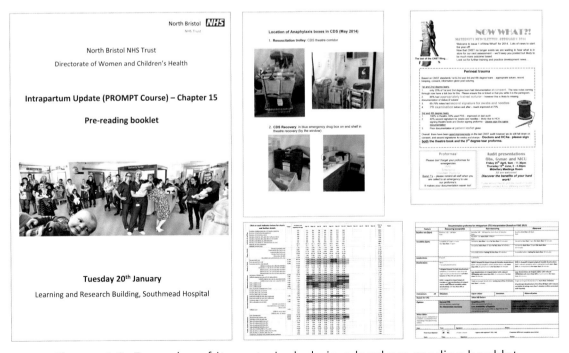

Figure 1.2 Examples of items to include in a local pre-reading booklet

All presentations, handouts, equipment and props can be stored in a central location. It is useful if all the trainers are familiar with each other's workstations and lectures, so that they can interchange between stations when necessary. Equipment can be stored in plastic boxes (see Section 2: *Practical advice for facilitating drills and workshops*), which should be re-stocked at the end of each training session.

Multi-professional faculty and attendees

Current evidence supports training for obstetric emergencies in multi-professional teams for 100% of staff.[1,2,3] The key features of training programmes associated with improvements in perinatal outcome are:

- Training conducted in-house
- Training all maternity staff together
- 100% of maternity staff trained annually
- Incorporating teamwork principles into clinical training scenarios
- Introducing system changes, often suggested by their own staff after participating in the training

These key elements should be emphasised. Achieving optimal attendance requires the commitment and dedication of the whole unit and should be supported by both the midwifery and the medical leads in the department. It requires local 'champions' to maintain the momentum and to monitor whether local improvements have been achieved.

The recent NHS England Maternity Review, *Better Births*, recognises the benefits of local multi-professional training, recommending that *'those who work together should train together.'* Furthermore, they recommend that training, both for routine situations and emergencies, should be a standard part of continuous professional development.[4]

Course evaluation and certificates

There is no assessment form included in the PROMPT course materials, as PROMPT courses are for training staff and not for assessing staff competencies. We believe that individual pass/fail course assessments may do more harm than good: none of the testing has any predictive validity, and it is difficult to identify a robust threshold for success. In addition, if formal assessments were included, this might deter staff from attending the training day and also distract them from gaining whatever knowledge is appropriate for them. We use unit-based clinical outcome data to determine success rates, and have developed an automated and statistically informed dashboard to provide intrapartum outcomes from standard maternity databases (see *Course Manual* Module 16: Measuring quality in maternity care).

We have included course evaluation/feedback sheets for participants, which can provide very useful feedback about any systems or documentation that may have been piloted. Example certificates of attendance can also be printed from the downloadable supporting materials (see Appendix 2). They should be signed by the local training team.

References

1.   Draycott T, Sibanda T, Owen L, *et al.* Does training in obstetric emergencies improve neonatal outcome? *BJOG* 2006; 113: 177–82.

2.   Draycott T, Crofts J, Ash JP, *et al.* Improving neonatal outcome through practical shoulder dystocia training. *Obstet Gynecol* 2008; 112: 14–20.

3.   Siassakos D, Crofts JF, Winter C, Weiner CP, Draycott TJ. The active components of effective training in obstetric emergencies. *BJOG* 2009; 116: 1028–32.

4.   National Maternity Review. *Better Births: Improving Outcomes of Maternity Services in England*. London: NHS England, 2016.

Section 2
Practical advice for facilitating drills and workshops

Each obstetric emergency scenario/workshop includes:

- ■ Key learning points and common difficulties observed from previous drills
- ■ Scenario outline
- ■ Equipment lists
- ■ Aims of the scenario
- ■ Drill facilitator instructions – including handover and drill prompts
- ■ Patient-actor script and instructions
- ■ Maternity notes, partogram (where appropriate), charts and documentation pro formas
- ■ Treatment algorithms
- ■ Clinical and teamwork checklists to facilitate debriefing
- ■ PowerPoint lectures and commentaries
- ■ Some workshops also include demonstration videos

Introduction

The scenarios included in this 3rd edition of the *Trainer's Manual* have been designed to enable teams of midwives, obstetricians, anaesthetists, maternity care assistants and other maternity care providers to practise managing some of the rare but potentially life-threatening obstetric emergencies that may occur in hospital, in a midwife-led birth centre or at home. The scenarios are not complicated and outline only the immediate emergency actions required, but can easily be made more complex or adapted to emphasise specific points from real-life cases that have occurred in your unit or institution.

Participation in simulated drills can be a nerve-wracking experience for some healthcare professionals, and this is often the first challenge to be met. Over time, participants usually overcome their initial embarrassment and appreciate the opportunity to practise managing emergencies in simulated circumstances with other members of their maternity teams.

Key learning points and difficulties observed

At the beginning of each section we have listed key learning points that trainers should aim to achieve. We have also included common difficulties that we have observed when running previous drills which may assist the trainers when facilitating the scenarios, and can also help to guide the debrief sessions afterwards.

'Ice-breaker'

The course programme starts with an introductory session and a team activity, an 'ice-breaker', which is designed to help the participants get to know each other and introduce the concept of team communication and teamworking. There are two 'ice-breaker' activities to choose from in Section 5 of this manual.

Enthusiasm

Our past experience of running interactive training drills has identified the importance of an enthusiastic and supportive approach from all trainers. Participants should be made to feel welcome and relaxed in this unfamiliar setting. This is vital to the success of the course.

Scenario realism

Where possible, the scenarios are best undertaken in the relevant clinical area to ensure the highest environmental fidelity: e.g. labour ward (including birth centre and pool rooms), maternal critical care rooms, or other appropriate clinical areas such as obstetric theatres for the anaesthetic/

theatre scenarios. However, if clinical rooms are not free on the day, then offices or similar rooms may be used, aided by the use of simple props to encourage realism (see **Appendix 3**).

Using a patient-actor, or using a patient-actor in combination with a mannequin, can also increase the realism of the scenario and enhance the communication between team members and the woman. It can also be useful for the patient-actor to give feedback 'from a woman's perspective' after each drill.

A member of staff who has had previous experience of being involved in the particular emergency being portrayed can make an excellent patient-actor. Alternatively, asking healthcare assistants to be the patient-actor may be an effective way of giving them insight into how the multi-professional team might manage the emergency, and at the same time it may help to reduce the anxiety that staff sometimes feel about participating in simulated scenarios.

Where a full-body mannequin is used in some of the scenarios, we have suggested that one of the trainers could play the birth partner, thus encouraging participants to communicate with the partner as well.

Equipment and training mannequins

If drills are to be run well, the correct equipment should be available, and equipment lists are provided with each scenario. Equipment can be stored in a central location in separate plastic boxes with contents lists attached inside the lid to facilitate easy stocking up after use (Figure 2.1).

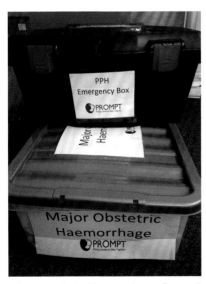 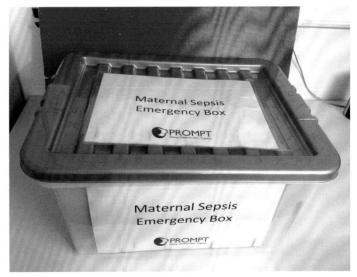

Figure 2.1 Examples of equipment boxes

There is also increasing evidence of improvements in outcomes related to the use of specific training mannequins; in particular the PROMPT Birthing Trainer was identified as a common theme in a number of successful training programmes for shoulder dystocia, and is recognised in the RCOG Green-top Guideline (2012).[1]

Scenario props

We have developed some very simple but helpful props to increase the realism of the scenarios, such as 'bloodstained' incontinence sheets, 'magic trousers' that bleed and a 'magic cushion' to use for the inverted uterus. We have also included example photographs of clinical equipment, which can be downloaded, laminated and used if non-clinical rooms need to be used (see Appendix 3). Ideally, we would encourage you to take photos of your own emergency bells and equipment, so that staff become familiar with the appearance of their own equipment.

Emergency boxes and trolleys

Training days provide the opportunity for staff to familiarise themselves with the contents and location of their emergency boxes or trolleys. It is important that any emergency boxes or trolleys used on the training day are exactly the same as the emergency equipment used in the clinical area, and if possible it should be located in the actual place too. In addition, the system for ensuring that boxes/trolleys are stocked after use can be discussed during the sessions, so that all staff are aware of this system. The emergency boxes should contain a treatment algorithm, and staff should be encouraged to allocate one member of the team to read out the separate treatment steps during the scenarios, as they are recommended to do in the real emergencies.

Prompting during drills/scenarios

The drill facilitator running each scenario needs to be willing to prompt the participants at certain times, such as when they freeze or are unsure of what to do next. Gentle prompting can relieve the situation and get the scenario back on the right track. There is little educational benefit in allowing someone to flounder and feel humiliated in their struggle to manage a situation.

There is, however, a fine line between helping and interfering. Where possible, the scenarios should be allowed to run with the drill facilitator acting only as an observer and occasional prompter. It may also be appropriate to allow the team to make errors or omissions during the drill, as long as these are identified and discussed in the post-drill debriefing session.

Record keeping

Documenting the actions taken during the simulated drills is as important as the management of the emergencies themselves. A set of maternity notes and (where appropriate) a partogram can be printed off and used to aid the handover of the scenario in the labour ward room. These can also act as a reminder of the woman's history and can be used to document the subsequent care given during the scenario. You may prefer to make up your own notes and partograms using local paperwork. An example of a MOEWS chart (Modified Obstetric Early Warning Score chart), a maternal critical care chart and an SBAR (situation, background, assessment, recommendation) handover sheet can all be printed from the downloadable materials and used during the scenarios. However, we would encourage the use of local observation charts where possible, as this is a good way of ensuring that staff are familiar with their local charts, and also useful for piloting new charts and aiding the implementation of new systems on 'the shop floor'.

In addition, there are structured documentation pro formas provided for some of the drill scenarios and fetal monitoring workshops, which can be adapted for clinical use in your own unit or institution.

It is a good idea to suggest that the team allocate the role of scribe to one person during each drill. The importance of accurate documentation should always be stressed in the post-drill discussions.

Drill briefing

It can be useful to include a drill briefing for the participants at the start of the simulation session, to clarify exactly what actions the participants should undertake during the drills. For example, if you would like them to actually draw up the medications or move the bed out of the room, then explain this before the drill starts. Important safety information should also be included in the briefing.

Listed below are some instructions that you may find useful to read out. They can be amended as necessary to suit your local circumstances:

- Please carry out all the actions you would normally do.

- When calling for help, pretend to use the call bell or emergency buzzer and then state clearly the help you require.

- Always use the 'needleless' intravenous cannulae provided, when required.

- IV fluids may be run through giving sets and attached to the cannulae, but do not actually start them flowing. (Or specify if you want them to use previously prepared fluids, to be more economical, or photographs of fluid bags etc.)

- If appropriate, go through the motions of taking blood by using the appropriate blood bottles, labelling them, completing the blood forms and saying where they should be sent. (This may also be important if there have been any risk issues identified by the blood transfusion department, such as incorrect labelling of blood bottles.)

- Obtain and draw up any medication that you need to use (or simulated vials if using these).

- Simulate administering the medication by the appropriate route, but do not use any sharps.

- Attach any equipment you would normally use; for example, if you wish to take someone's blood pressure, attach the cuff and ask the facilitator for the reading.

- If you need additional information, you may ask the facilitator during the scenario.

- Please take care with the patient-actors – just as you would for anyone receiving maternity care.

It can also be helpful, before each scenario, to orientate participants to the equipment and the area in which the scenario is taking place. We have found that participants are able to relax and better immerse themselves in the teaching if they are told:

- Where? Where is this drill taking place? (This is especially important if it is not taking place in the clinical environment.)

- What? What emergency equipment has been made available for them, and where is it located?

- How? How should they interact with the mannequin/patient-actor? How will you as facilitator be running the scenario? How can they obtain help if they need it? How are they expected to draw up drugs, measure vital signs, etc. during *this* scenario?

■ **Who?** Who is participating, and who is observing? (i.e. assign roles)

■ The participants should then be given an opportunity to ask any questions.

Participants who are appropriately briefed are less likely to be stressed, more likely to enjoy the drill, and will thereby gain more learning.

Team to be trained

A sensible size for the multi-professional team participating in the drill is six to eight people. With programmes 1 and 2, where the format is lecture/drill/lecture, it may be useful to allocate two teams to each of the scenarios. One team can participate in the drill before the lecture while the other team observes, and then they can swap over for the repeat drill after the lecture. Obviously, this means that the team participating in the drill after the lecture will have a double advantage in that they have not only watched the other team perform first but have also attended the lecture. However, if you alternate which team goes first for each of the different scenarios then they should all get a chance at being both the first and the second team.

One of the key reasons for including all members of the maternity team in the drill training is so that staff do not have to roleplay outside of their usual roles and can practise the specific actions required within their role, during each emergency. It also allows participants to become familiar with each other's roles. It may be helpful to give participants self-adhesive labels to wear during the scenario so that it is easy to identify roles within each team (e.g. typed labels with Midwife, Anaesthetist, Junior Obstetrician, Senior Obstetrician etc.). There is a template for printing off various staff-role labels included in the downloadable materials.

The scenario handover

We have found it works well to take one member of the team into the room first for a handover, while the rest of the team waits outside. The patient-actor scripts have been designed so that the emergency occurs after about half a minute, thus prompting initial action from the first team member in the room. By doing this, the original team member also has to state the problem clearly to the other team members as they arrive to help, thus emphasising the importance of this initial action.

Participants should be asked to **pretend** to use the call bell or emergency alarm, as appropriate, and to state which other team members they would like to attend to help them.

It is worth considering alternating which participant takes the handover, so that the same participant is not always the first on the scene. Some participants may be nervous or reluctant to be the first on the scene; participants should be encouraged, but not coerced, into full participation in the drills.

It may be more realistic to send the help requested into the room after a period of 20–30 seconds, rather than straight away, as assistance does not always arrive immediately in real life. The few seconds between calling for help and the staff members arriving can be quite frightening, but is it is also the time when essential emergency actions such as lowering the bed head, moving the woman to left-lateral position, opening the airway and administering oxygen are required. It is, however, reassuring for the participant to be told that help is on the way, particularly if he or she appears anxious.

Clinical and teamwork checklists

There are specific clinical and teamwork checklists provided to help to structure observation of clinical actions and components of team working during the drills. If there are enough people, one or two members of the participating team, or of the observing team, if there are two teams for each scenario, should observe the drill and complete the checklists. The checklists can provide a useful starting point for debriefing after the scenario.

The three key components of team working are: communication; team roles and responsibilities; and situational awareness. These components are integrated into the scenarios using the teamwork checklists. There is a teamwork powerpoint presentation explaining these three teamwork components in more detail, included in the *Course introduction and teamwork* presentation (see **Section 4**: *Team working and teamwork training*).

Giving feedback after drills/scenarios

On completion of each drill there should be a debrief session, the depth and detail of which will be determined by the amount of time available. Those participating in the drill often perceive that they have performed very badly, so it is vital that positive actions are emphasised during the debrief session.

Giving feedback after simulation is one of the most powerful influences on learning and achievement.[2] In a synthesis of over 800 meta-analyses, simulation training which included a feedback session was found to have double the effect, compared to simulation alone.[3] However, individual approaches to giving feedback vary in their effectiveness, making the overall impact either positive or negative.[4]

Elements of effective feedback

Feedback is most effective if it:

- Focuses on the task not the learner
- Can be elaborated upon
- Is presented in manageable units
- Has specific and clear messages
- Is as simple as possible
- Reduces uncertainty between performance and goals
- Is unbiased and objective, written or via computer if possible
- Promotes learning through goal orientation
- Is provided after learners have attempted a solution

There are several methods of giving feedback.[5] One popular method, the 'hamburger' method (positive, negative, positive; a.k.a. Pendleton's rules), is now considered one of the least effective. More recently, other techniques have been suggested.

We have chosen one simple method which aims to encourage the team to discuss their thoughts and feelings on how they felt the drill went, and also to prompt them to suggest ways that they could improve it. The observations of the facilitator(s), and feedback from the observers who have been completing the clinical and teamwork checklists, should also be given. If the scenario includes a patient-actor, that person too can comment on the team's performance. Finally, group discussion should be encouraged, including suggestions from the team about system improvements that may have been identified as a result of running the drill/scenario.

To help structure the feedback session, the trainers may ask the participants four key questions, as follows:

1. 'How do you feel that went?'

This creates 'buy-in' and commits the participants to accept their performance as their own. It can also give you an opportunity to gauge the level of insight the participants have into their own performance. They may use this opportunity to vent emotions about the drill/scenario or even about how it was set up; if they do, acknowledge these feelings sympathetically. This will allow the emotions to be put to one side, so that the team can concentrate on learning.

2. 'What do you think you did effectively?'

This question on its own doesn't help the participants, but it does make them more receptive to what will follow. It is also an opportunity to highlight and reinforce particularly effective actions or behaviours. You can then repeat this question to those feeding back from the clinical and teamwork checklists, as well as the patient-actor.

3. 'What would you do differently next time?'

Participants are more likely to be receptive to self-identified areas for improvement. Build on these if you can. It is vital to help participants identify areas for improvement and a realistic way of achieving them (see *Elements of effective feedback*, above). For example, participants may identify that 'communication' could be improved, but are unsure how to improve it. Based on your observations, you may suggest that in the next drill/scenario, someone declares the emergency, utilises eye contact, or uses 'closed-loop' communication. Afterwards, this question can then be put to those feeding back from the checklists, and any patient-actor.

4. 'Would you like me to tell you how you could improve?'

Hopefully you won't need to get to this question, if the participants have already identified areas for improvement and also methods for improving themselves. If not, focus on providing realistic goals and ways that they can help to achieve them.

There is a video demonstration of how to set up and run a **maternal sepsis drill** included in the downloadable supporting materials. It also provides additional suggestions on how the trainers may facilitate and debrief after the drill.

Running hands-on practical workshops

For some simulated emergencies, we suggest that the session may be run as a 'hands-on' practical workshop instead of a simulated drill. This works particularly well for the shoulder dystocia session, where it is beneficial for all team members to gain hands-on experience of the internal manoeuvres. If there is sufficient time then it may be possible to run a hands-on session followed by a simulated scenario to reinforce the learning. Whether the session is just a hands-on workshop or a drill, the training team should still encourage feedback and discussion from all team members, and include relevant aspects of team working and documentation.

There is also a demonstration video on how to run a hands-on practical workshop for the management of **shoulder dystocia** included in the downloadable training materials.

References

1. Royal College of Obstetricians and Gynaecologists. *Shoulder Dystocia*, 2nd edn. Green-top Guideline No. 42. London: RCOG, 2012. www.rcog.org.uk/en/guidelines-research-services/guidelines/gtg42 (accessed August 2017).

2. Hattie J, Timperley H. The power of feedback. *Review of Educational Research* 2007; 77: 81–112. DOI: 10.3102/003465430298487.

3. Hattie J. *Visible Learning: a Synthesis of Over 800 Meta-Analyses Relating to Achievement*. Abingdon: Routledge, 2008.

4. Shute VJ. *Focus on Formative Feedback*. ETS Research and Development RR-07-11. Educational Testing Service, 2007. www.ets.org/Media/Research/pdf/RR-07-11.pdf (accessed August 2017).

5. For example, see Cantillon P, Sargeant J. Giving feedback in clinical settings. *BMJ* 2008; 337: a1961.

Section 3
Local PROMPT implementation

Training for obstetric emergencies is not always effective. Currently, the evidence supports annual, local multi-professional training, with integrated teamwork/human factors elements, for all maternity staff.[1]

PROMPT is an evidence-based programme for the entire multi-professional maternity team that should be implemented locally. Using practice-based tools, workshops and emergency drills with simple props, clinical algorithms, high-fidelity mannequins and patient-actors, PROMPT aims to optimise the management of obstetric emergencies.[2]

Attending a PROMPT T3 programme is just the start; hopefully, it will be a great start and will leave your team brimming with enthusiasm to get PROMPT introduced in your local setting. However, we recognise that local implementation can sometimes be challenging, and we have therefore put together some tips and advice gained from our experience of implementing PROMPT at scale, in Australia and Scotland.

Successful implementation is considered to have four elements:[3]

1. External environment – e.g. policy landscape, government initiatives, funding etc.
2. Structure of the organisation – e.g. local and regional context and support
3. Characteristics of the innovation – core elements of PROMPT, versus peripheral elements
4. Processes used – local integration, including management buy-in and support

Clearly all of these elements are linked, and indeed they need to be aligned and joined up for an authentic implementation of PROMPT that will improve perinatal outcomes.

The PROMPT course is designed to be adapted locally across many different settings. It is often said that *'PROMPT provides the bricks, for local units to build their own house.'* However, it is equally important that teams understand and follow the building regulations to ensure that they build a robust, sustainable PROMPT programme locally. One of the key issues is an understanding of the elements of PROMPT that are core and need to be implemented in full for maximum effect, compared to those elements that are more peripheral and may usefully be adapted at local level.[4]

Shoulder dystocia training appears to be one of these core elements, where reductions in brachial plexus injury are associated with training programmes that use the RCOG (PROMPT) shoulder dystocia algorithm and the PROMPT mannequin (Limbs & Things). It does not seem to be helpful to use mnemonics instead of the algorithm,[5] and their use has been associated with either no change in brachial plexus injury after training,[6,7] or even increases in poor outcomes.[8] Local training is not cheap,[9] and therefore it is vital that maternity units implement effective, evidence-based training. Most importantly, it is a tragedy for the individuals whose injury could have been prevented. There is also evidence of differences in outcomes related to the use of different training mannequins; the PROMPT mannequin was a common theme in a number of successful training programmes,[10,11] as is recognised in the RCOG guideline: *'Shoulder dystocia training associated with improvements in clinical management and neonatal outcomes was multi-professional, with manoeuvres demonstrated and practised on a high fidelity mannequin. Teaching used the RCOG algorithm rather than staff being taught mnemonics (e.g. HELPERR) or eponyms (e.g. Rubin's and Woods' screw).'*[12]

While we recommend that PROMPT training should be based on national guidance and recommendations, it can be very useful to localise certain peripheral elements to more accurately reflect local practice. Making videos with local staff can also help to illustrate elements of team working and local care differences.

One significant difficulty for units is the cost of sustaining local training programmes. It is not cheap, and 92% of the cost is staff time.[9] It is essential that unit-level managers are engaged with the potential benefits of training – harnessing national initiatives and financial incentives[13] with returns in the form of reduced litigation payments[10,11,13,14,15] and improved staff safety attitudes.[16] A business case for training can be developed with your local PROMPT trainers.

Initiative fatigue can also be an issue,[17] particularly given the current plethora of safety initiatives raining down from central government. Moreover, there can also be confusion over the many tools and processes used by different parts of the maternity team: a common mistake when introducing new practices is to add another set of tools (e.g. stickers/mnemonics for CTGs) on top of the existing ones, which only serves to divide and confuse staff. Once again, it is useful for all staff in one department/unit to use a single evidence-based system, and it is vital that they train together to learn how to use it, i.e. in communities of practice.[18]

Finally, there can be additional challenges due to insufficient support for local training teams when they are trying to develop and implement their in-house PROMPT courses. Provisional findings from the THISTLE-Plus study (a parallel process study investigating the implementation of PROMPT in maternity units in Scotland) are that staff would like more support, particularly in some of the smaller units that may have less capacity for training, or those units that are new to running local training programmes. Similar findings have been reported by other non-maternity safety initiatives.[18] A very successful innovation promoted by the Victorian Managed Insurance Authority (VMIA) in Australia is the use of quarterly meetings for the local PROMPT champions from all of the units currently running PROMPT in the state of Victoria. PROMPT has been successfully implemented in Victoria, with significant improvements in perinatal outcomes.[19] However, the units valued the opportunity to meet and share challenges and solutions, as well as new innovations. There were also buddying opportunities for newer units embarking on PROMPT training and 6-monthly refreshers with new drills shared across the region.

Another Australian innovation is a networked approach to supporting local training, as used in West Gippsland. This is a very rural part of the state of Victoria with a number of very small maternity units (80–1000 births per annum) where a central PROMPT faculty works with the smaller units, including local general practitioners, midwives, nurses and emergency department staff, to facilitate local training.

Hopefully we have given your teams a few ideas that may make the implementation process a little smoother, and we wish you every success with your local PROMPT programme. We have enhanced the *10 steps to successful PROMPT implementation* that were recommended in the second edition of the PROMPT training package, and we hope these will provide you with an excellent place to start. Additional support and resources are also available from the PROMPT Maternity Foundation team to aid your local PROMPT implementation (info@promptmaternity.org).

The 10 steps to successful PROMPT implementation

1. Multi-professional participants, trainers and drills
2. Locally run courses in your own unit, using your own facilities and training **all** your maternity staff annually
3. Integrated team working within the clinical sessions
4. Locally adopted and adapted training (must remain in line with national guidance)
5. Support from midwifery and medical management and in-house clinical 'champions'
6. Use of simple props and patient-actors
7. Use of the PROMPT Birthing Trainer and PROMPT (RCOG) algorithm for shoulder dystocia
8. Include testing and implementation of new local systems and protocols within training
9. Participant debriefing following drills, using clinical and teamwork checklists
10. Monitoring and evaluation of local clinical outcomes

References

1. Draycott TJ, Collins KJ, Crofts JF, *et al.* Myths and realities of training in obstetric emergencies. *Best Pract Res Clin Obstet Gynaecol* 2015; 29: 1067–76.

2. National Maternity Review. *Better Births: Improving Outcomes of Maternity Services in England*. London: NHS England, 2016.

3. Fisher ES, Shortell SM, Savitz LA. Implementation science: a potential catalyst for delivery system reform. *JAMA* 2016; 315: 339–40.

4. Haynes A, Brennan S, Redman S, *et al.*; CIPHER Team. Figuring out fidelity: a worked example of the methods used to identify, critique and revise the essential elements of a contextualised intervention in health policy agencies. *Implement Sci* 2016; 11(1): 23. www.ncbi.nlm.nih.gov/pmc/articles/PMC4765223 (accessed August 2017).

5. Jan H, Guimicheva B, Gosh S, *et al.* Evaluation of healthcare professionals' understanding of eponymous maneuvers and mnemonics in emergency obstetric care provision. *Int J Gynaecol Obstet* 2014; 125: 228–31.

6. Walsh JM, Kandamany N, Ni Shuibhne N, *et al.* Neonatal brachial plexus injury: comparison of incidence and antecedents between 2 decades. *Am J Obstet Gynecol* 2011; 204: 324.e1–6.

7. Fransen AF, van de Ven J, Schuit E, *et al.* Simulation-based team training for multi-professional obstetric care teams to improve patient outcome: a multicentre, cluster randomised controlled trial. *BJOG* 2017; 124: 641–50.

8. MacKenzie I, Shah M, Lean K, *et al.* Management of shoulder dystocia: trends in incidence and maternal and neonatal morbidity. *Obstet Gynecol* 2007; 110: 1059–68.

9. Yau CW, Pizzo E, Morris S, *et al.* The cost of local, multi-professional obstetric emergencies training. *Acta Obstet Gynecol Scand* 2016; 95: 1111–19.

10. Weiner CP, Collins L, Bentley S, Dong Y, Satterwhite CL. Multi-professional training for obstetric emergencies in a U.S. hospital over a 7-year interval: an observational study. *J Perinatol* 2016; 36: 19–24.

11. Crofts J, Lenguerrand E, Bentham GL, *et al.* Prevention of brachial plexus injury: 12 years of shoulder dystocia training: an interrupted time-series study. *BJOG* 2016; 123: 111–18.

12. Royal College of Obstetricians and Gynaecologists. *Shoulder Dystocia*, 2nd edn. Green-top Guideline No. 42. London: RCOG, 2012. www.rcog.org.uk/en/guidelines-research-services/guidelines/gtg42 (accessed August 2017).

13. Sagar R, Draycott T, Hogg S. The role of insurers in maternity safety. *Best Pract Res Clin Obstet Gynaecol* 2015; 29: 1126–31.

14. Pettker CM, Thung SF, Lipkind HS, *et al.* A comprehensive obstetric patient safety program reduces liability claims and payments. *Am J Obstet Gynecol* 2014; 211: 319–25.

15. Riley W, Meredith LW, Price R, et al. Decreasing malpractice claims by reducing preventable perinatal harm. *Health Serv Res* 2016; 51(Suppl 3): 2453–71.

16. Siassakos D, Fox R, Hunt L, *et al.* Attitudes toward safety and teamwork in a maternity unit with embedded team training. *Am J Med Qual* 2011; 26: 132–7.

17. Pannick S, Sevdalis N, Athanasiou T. Beyond clinical engagement: a pragmatic model for quality improvement interventions, aligning clinical and managerial priorities. *BMJ Qual Saf* 2016; 25: 716–25.

18. Dixon-Woods M, Bosk CL, Aveling EL, Goeschel CA, Pronovost PJ. Explaining Michigan: developing an ex post theory of a quality improvement program. *Milbank Q* 2011; 89: 167–205.

19. Shoushtarian M, Barnett M, McMahon F, Ferris J. Impact of introducing practical obstetric multi-professional training (PROMPT) into maternity units in Victoria, Australia. *BJOG* 2014; 121: 1710–18.

Section 4
Team working and teamwork training

Key learning points

- Good team working is important, because poorly functioning teams are associated with preventable harm for mothers and babies.
- More efficient teams state the emergency earlier and use closed-loop communication.
- Teamwork training, when incorporated into clinical training, is associated with improvements in clinical outcomes.
- Effective teams appreciate the different roles and responsibilities of team members and the importance of shared decision making. They are also able to 'stand back and take a broader view' in an emergency situation.
- Multi-professional training locally for all staff has been associated with improved teamwork, improved safety attitudes and, most importantly, improved perinatal outcomes.
- For these reasons, recent national reports recommend that teams that work together should also train together.

Problems identified with local training

- Not training all groups and grades of staff together
- Not incorporating teamwork training into clinical training
- Staff working in 'silos' and not understanding the value of shared decision making

Introduction

Poor team working is directly associated with preventable harm for mothers and babies, with poor communication and team working identified as major contributors in the MBRRACE-UK Report (2014).[1] There have been repeated recommendations for more, and better, teamwork training in national reports,[1,2,3] and, more recently, for 'human factors training'.[4] However, a number of studies have demonstrated that isolated team working and/or human factors training do not appear to be associated with improvements in clinical[5,6] or process[7] outcomes. Therefore, it is important to understand and implement only those team training interventions that have been shown to be clinically effective, particularly for maternity teams.[8]

In one study of simulated eclampsia,[8] the most efficient maternity teams:

- stated (recognised and verbally declared) the emergency earlier
- used closed-loop communication (task clearly delegated, accepted, executed and completion acknowledged)
- had significantly fewer exits from the labour room (related to improved communication)
- used a structured form of communication (such as SBAR)

Integrating and teaching these team behaviours within simulated emergency drills has been associated with improved outcomes in both the UK and the US.[8,9,10]

Improving team working is important, and the current evidence base supports local, multi-professional training for all staff annually, with teamwork training integrated into clinical training.[11]

Teamwork themes

For this third edition of the PROMPT training package, we have continued with the three key teamwork themes that have been demonstrated to be important in obstetric simulation and during category 1 emergency births.[8,12,13]

The key teamwork themes are:

- Communication
- Team roles and leadership
- Situational awareness – 'standing back and taking a broader view'

These three interrelated themes are integrated throughout the course programme. There are some teamwork slides included within the *Course introduction and teamwork* presentation, and there are teamwork checklists included in each of the drill scenarios.

The main features to be considered for each theme are:

- **Communication** should be:
    - ☐ clearly worded – a clear message
    - ☐ addressed, with specific instructions directed to an appropriate team member
    - ☐ sent in a clear and timely manner
    - ☐ heard and acknowledged
    - ☐ understood and checked back for verification
- When observing **team roles and leadership**, a good team member will:
    - ☐ have a specified, clearly understood role (including a leader)
    - ☐ be adaptable and flexible
    - ☐ assume responsibility for their actions
    - ☐ feel comfortable enough to advocate
    - ☐ feed back information to the rest of the team in a timely fashion
    - ☐ be mutually supportive
- The features of **situational awareness** (standing back and taking a broader view):
    - ☐ **Notice**: be aware of the woman's condition and evaluate if treatment is being effective
    - ☐ Also consider each team member and available resources
    - ☐ Assess how the team are coping and anticipate potential errors by noticing cues and cross-checking with team members
    - ☐ **Understand**: share information with the team, think what these cues and clues may mean, be aware of common pitfalls, re-evaluate/stand back at regular intervals, seek to engage team members in decisions
    - ☐ **Think ahead**: continually re-evaluate, anticipate, plan and prioritise

Using teamwork checklists during debrief

Debriefing methods are reviewed in Section 2, including the use of teamwork checklists to aid the debriefing process after a simulated drill. There is evidence that allocating observers to use the teamwork checklists to comment on their own team's behaviour in the drills is associated with improved decision-to-birth intervals and neonatal outcomes during real-life emergencies.[8]

Therefore we have used teamwork checklists to structure team debriefing sessions following drills/scenarios, and to reinforce the key teamwork and communication messages. The checklists can usefully be printed off and laminated for repeated use during drills (they are included in the downloadable supporting materials, incorporated within the specific folder for each clinical emergency). At the end of each scenario in this manual we have included one or more checklists, selecting those themes of team working that are most likely to be relevant to the specific emergency. However, any combination of the teamwork checklists may be used, according to local preference. The three different teamwork checklists are shown below.

During the Training the Trainers (T3) programme the trainers will share some examples of film clips that can be used to help demonstrate some of these teamwork themes. We have also produced some videos of simulated drills that can be viewed by participants so that they can identify key aspects of communication and team working.

Teamwork checklists

Teamwork checklist: communication

Communication		YES	NO
State the problem	Clinical problem was stated clearly to arriving team		
Instructions	Instructions were clearly worded		
	Unnecessary conversation/noise was avoided		
	Action plans were shared		
	Goals were clearly identified		
Addressed	Specific instructions were given to the appropriate team members		
Sent	Communication was not rushed		
	It was clear what action was required		
Heard	Acknowledgements were made		
	Requests for repeat information were made		
Understood	The information was understood and repeated back by recipient		
	The correct action was performed		

Teamwork checklist: team roles and leadership

Team roles and leadership		YES	NO
Roles	Each team member had a clear role		
	There was a team leader		
Adaptability	Team members responded well to different situations		
Responsibility	Team members assumed responsibility for their role		
Advocate	Tasks were delegated appropriately		
Feedback	There were regular updates on progress		
	A running commentary was provided		
Support	Team members did not argue about issues		
	None of the team members decided to 'go it alone'		

Teamwork checklist: situational awareness

Situational awareness/standing back, taking a broader view		YES	NO
Notice	There was an awareness of what each member of the team was doing		
	There was an awareness of the resources that were needed		
	Mistakes were identified		
Understand	Regular updates took place throughout the scenario		
	Problems were identified		
	A re-evaluation was undertaken		
	Team members were asked for their opinion		
	Team members were asked to suggest possible solutions		
	A clear action plan was made		
Prioritise	Key tasks were given priority		
Delegate	Each team member had a specific task		
	The tasks were delegated appropriately		

Safety checklists

Recently, safety checklists have become a ubiquitous part of preparation for surgery. Although their use has been adopted for obstetric interventions, some adaptation is required for maternity care.[14] Obstetric surgery is most often performed under regional anaesthesia, and frequently there is a birth partner present too, meaning that good communication with the woman and her partner must continue throughout the procedure; this is quite different from surgery performed under general anaesthesia. Many units have therefore adapted the safety checklist to include the mother and her partner in the questions on the checklist, i.e. the team is introduced to the mother, rather than to each other, and the mother is directly asked to confirm the operation and her allergies, etc. Directing the questions to the mother and including her birth partner has been demonstrated to improve how reassured they both feel, as well as to enhance their post-birth satisfaction (personal communication, Catherine Simmonds).[15] Women and their birth partners could, and should, be included as part of the birth team. An example of a safety checklist for maternity theatres is included in the downloadable materials.

A *maternal critical care review sheet* is another example of a safety checklist that provides a structured approach to the frequent multi-professional reviews required for a pregnant or postnatal woman who is critically ill. A copy is included in Section 13.

Handover of care

Handover is also a key part of team working and communication. As part of a Health Foundation-supported maternity project, we investigated labour ward handovers using a validated observation tool.

Although the handovers were perceived to be very effective by the clinicians, an independent review by non-clinical members of staff identified problems with:

- introducing team members and roles (46% poor or no introduction)
- numerous interruptions during the handover, which hampered the transfer of information
- formulating action plans (53% poor allocation or no action plan)

After sharing these findings with all maternity staff on the labour ward (clinical and non-clinical), the staff spontaneously suggested improvements to the handover:

- All team members should introduce themselves and their roles at the beginning of the handover.
- Reduce interruptions to a minimum by:
  - □ placing a 'handover in progress' sign on the door
  - □ midwife coordinator to give drug cupboard keys to outside staff
  - □ staff attending the handover only to be called out if there is an emergency call
- Adopt a more structured method for communicating information (e.g. use of SBAR).
- Continue to nurture an open environment.

A '*key points for labour ward handover*' sheet was produced, which all staff could refer to. A video demonstrating the format for the revised labour ward handover and safety briefing was also made. Both of these are included in the downloadable materials.

In many ways the labour ward board round is the UK equivalent of the 'team huddles' described in some US settings, with many similar positives.[16] Clearly, labour ward handover often occurs at the start of a shift, but these positive behaviours should be continuous throughout the shift, and should include communication with the woman and her family.

SBAR

It has been established that the most effective maternity teams use a structured SBAR-style method of communication (situation, background, assessment, recommendation/response) (Figure 4.1).

The SBAR chart has also been very popular with community midwifery staff when referring women into the labour ward from home, as it has helped them structure and focus essential clinical information required by the receiving team.

We have included the use of an obstetric-specific SBAR chart in the maternal sepsis scenario (Section 11), which you can use to introduce and/or reinforce SBAR-style communication.

SBAR obstetric handover sheet for an urgent clinical situation

S

Situation

I am calling about (woman's name): _____ Ward: _____ Hosp No: _____

The problem I am calling about is: _____

I have just made an assessment:

Her vital signs are: Respirations_____ Blood pressure ____ /____ Pulse ____ SPO$_2$ _____% Temperature_____ ^{0}C

I am concerned about:

☐ **Respirations** because they are:
    ☐ less than 10
    ☐ over 30
    ☐ The woman is having oxygen at _____ l/min
☐ **Blood pressure** because it is:
    ☐ systolic over 160
    ☐ diastolic over 100
    ☐ systolic less than 90
☐ **Pulse** because it is:
    ☐ over 120
    ☐ less than 40

☐ **Urine output** because it is:
    ☐ less than 100 ml over the last 4 hours
    ☐ significantly proteinuric (+++)
☐ **Haemorrhage**:
    ☐ Antepartum
    ☐ Postpartum
☐ **Fetal wellbeing**:
    ☐ Fetal bradycardia
    ☐ Pathological CTG
☐ **FBS Result: pH** _____
    Time sample taken: _____ hrs

Obstetric Early Warning Chart Score:

B

Background (tick relevant sections)

The woman is:
    ☐ Nulliparous ☐ Multiparous ☐ Grand multiparous
    ☐ Gestation: _____ wks ☐ Singleton ☐ Multiple
    ☐ Previous Caesarean section or uterine surgery
☐ **Fetal wellbeing**
    ☐ Abdominal palpation:
    ☐ Fundal height:_____cm ☐ Presentation:_____ Fifths palpable: _____ FH rate:_____bpm
    ☐ Intrapartum CTG: ☐ Normal ☐ Suspicious ☐ Pathological
☐ **Antenatal**
    ☐ A/N Risk sheet (details): _____
    ☐ Antenatal CTG: ☐ Normal ☐ Abnormal
☐ **Labour**
    ☐ Spontaneous onset ☐ Induced
    ☐ IUGR ☐ Pre eclampsia ☐ Reduced fetal movements ☐ Diabetes ☐ APH
    ☐ Syntocinon infusion
    ☐ Most recent vaginal examination: Time _____hrs
    ☐ Cervical dilatation: _____cm ☐ Station of presenting part: _____ ☐ Position: _____
    ☐ Membranes ruptured ☐ Meconium stained liquor ☐ Fresh red loss PV
    ☐ Third stage complete ☐ Retained placenta
☐ **Birth details/post birth**
    ☐ Date of Birth: _____ Time of Birth:_____hrs
    ☐ Type of birth:_____ ☐ Perineal trauma:_____
    ☐ Blood loss: _____ml ☐ Syntocinon infusion
    ☐ Fundus: ☐ High ☐ Atonic ☐ Uterus tender ☐ Abdominal/perineal wound bleeding

A

Assessment

The problem seems to be: ☐ red flag sepsis ☐ cardiac ☐ respiratory ☐ haemorrhage
☐ severe PET ☐ HELLP ☐ pulmonary embolism ☐ pulmonary oedema ☐ severe fetal compromise
☐ I am not sure what the problem is, but the woman is deteriorating and we need to do something

☐ Treatment given / in progress:_____

R

Recommendation

Request:
☐ Please come to see the woman immediately
☐ I think delivering needs to be expedited
☐ I think the woman needs to be transferred to delivery suite
☐ I would like advice please

Reported to:_____ Response :_____

Person completing form (name):_____Date:_____ Time: _____

Figure 4.1 An example of an SBAR obstetric handover chart

References

1.   Knight M, Kenyon S, Brocklehurst P, *et al.* (eds.); MBRRACE-UK. *Saving Lives, Improving Mothers' Care: Lessons Learned to Inform Future Maternity Care from the UK and Ireland Confidential Enquiries into Maternal Deaths and Morbidity 2009–12*. Oxford: National Perinatal Epidemiology Unit, University of Oxford, 2014.

2.   Cantwell R, Clutton-Brock T, Cooper G, *et al.* Saving Mothers' Lives: reviewing maternal deaths to make motherhood safer: 2006–2008. The Eighth Report of the Confidential Enquiries into Maternal Deaths in the United Kingdom. *BJOG* 2011; 118 (Suppl. 1): 1–203.

3.   Institute of Medicine. *Crossing the Quality Chasm: A New Health System for the 21st Century*. Washington, DC: National Academies Press, 2001.

4.   Carthey J, Clarke J. *The 'How to Guide' for Implementing Human Factors in Healthcare*. Patient Safety First, 2009.

5.   Nielsen PE, Goldman MB, Mann S, *et al.* Effects of teamwork training on adverse outcomes and process of care in labor and delivery: a randomized controlled trial. *Obstet Gynecol* 2007; 109: 48–55.

6.   Timmons S, Baxendale B, Buttery A, *et al.* Implementing human factors in clinical practice. *Emerg Med J* 2015; 32: 368–72.

7.   Wears RL. Improvement and evaluation. *BMJ Qual Saf* 2015; 24: 92–4.

8.   Siassakos D, Hasafa Z, Sibanda T, *et al.* Retrospective cohort study of diagnosis–delivery interval with umbilical cord prolapse: the effect of team training. *BJOG* 2009; 116: 1089–96.

9.   Mann S, Pratt S. Role of clinician involvement in patient safety in obstetrics and gynecology. *Clin Obstet Gynecol* 2010; 53: 559–75.

10. Davis S, Riley W. Implementing and evaluating team training. *Jt Comm J Qual Patient Saf* 2011; 37: 339–40.

11. Draycott TJ, Collins KJ, Crofts JF, *et al.* Myths and realities of training in obstetric emergencies. *Best Pract Res Clin Obstet Gynaecol* 2015; 29: 1067–76.

12. Siassakos D, Bristowe K, Draycott T, *et al.* Clinical efficiency in a simulated emergency and relationship to team behaviours: a multisite cross-sectional study. *BJOG* 2011; 118: 596–607.

13. Siassakos D, Fox R, Crofts FJ, *et al.* The management of a simulated emergency: better team-work, better performance. *Resuscitation* 2011; 82: 203–6.

14. National Patient Safety Agency, Royal College of Obstetricians and Gynaecologists. The WHO surgical safety checklist: for maternity cases only, November 2010. www.nrls.npsa.nhs.uk /resources/?EntryId45=83972 (accessed August 2017).

15. Simmonds, C. Review of practice: facilitating normality at Caesarean section. *Journal of Perioperative Practice* 2016; 26 (7–8): 166–69.

16. Health Foundation. Using the huddle technique to improve patient safety, January 2015. www.health.org.uk/using-huddle-technique-improve-patient-safety (accessed August 2017).

Section 5
'Ice-breaker' team activities

Key learning points

■ To introduce team members to one another.
■ To introduce the three main themes of team working.

Introduction

There are two 'ice-breaker' activities included in this section. You may choose to use either one when running your PROMPT course:

■ Ice-breaker 1 is a practical task that engages all of the participants in each team (takes approximately 20 minutes).
■ Ice-breaker 2 is a team exercise requiring effective listening and communication skills (takes approximately 15–20 minutes).

There are PowerPoint slides which outline the instructions, rules and feedback for each ice-breaker activity included in the downloadable supporting materials.

Ice-breaker activity 1: build a tower

Aim

The aim of this activity is to encourage the participants to work together in their teams with a joint goal of building a tower. Run early in the day, this activity is a way of initiating effective communication and interaction within the team.

Equipment

Each multi-professional maternity unit team should be given the following equipment:

- 30 paper cups
- 30 cm masking tape
- 30 clothes pegs
- 2 PROMPT *Course Manuals*

Trainer's instructions

The trainer should ask each team to work together to build a tower using the materials provided and following the instructions below:

Specifications for tower

- Height at least 1.0 metres
- Use two *Course Manuals* within structure
- Should be floor-standing without using any additional support
- Only use materials provided

Planning phase – 5 minutes

Construction phase – 10 minutes

After the task

The trainers should review all of the towers and nominate a winning tower, which should be freestanding on the floor, have a height of over 1.0 metre and include two *Course Manuals* within the structure. You may even wish to award a prize for the best tower!

Figure 5.1 shows two examples of paper-cup towers, and more can be found in the online resources. These should not be shown to the students before they start, but can act as a guide for the faculty.

(a)   (b)

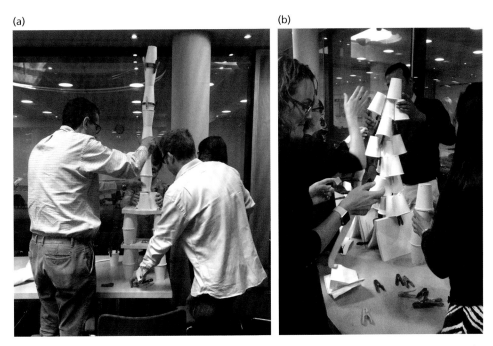

Figure 5.1 Examples of teams building a tower (ice-breaker activity 1)

Ice-breaker activity 2: draw a picture

Aim

Effective teamwork requires careful listening and clear communication. This activity requires the team to draw a predetermined picture, based only on limited oral instructions.

Learning objectives

- To be aware of the importance of listening carefully and responding to instructions
- To demonstrate differences in individual interpretation of information

Equipment

- One sheet of A4 paper per person
- One pencil/pen per person
- One picture to be described per team (from the downloadable materials)
- Blu-Tack to attach drawings to wall
- Teamwork checklists

Trainer's instructions

This activity is designed to test the communication and interpretation skills of the team members. It requires team members to reproduce a picture using only a verbal description and instructions given by one nominated team member, who can see the original picture. The likeness of the picture to the original will be determined by the communication and interpretation skills of the team members.

At the start of the task

Explain the task clearly and read out the rules of the exercise (see below). One nominated member from each team should be given a picture from the downloadable materials; they must not show the picture to the other members of the team. You may like to give all teams the same picture, so that the variation in the way the picture is described, and in the pictures produced, can be discussed, or you can give each team a different picture so that the resulting art gallery is more interesting. There are four different pictures included in the downloadable materials, and Figure 5.2 shows two examples.

Make sure the team cannot see the picture being described. If laminating the drawings, make sure you add an extra blank sheet behind the drawing before laminating, so that the picture cannot be seen through the back of the paper.

Nominate a describer and observer

Each team should nominate one member to describe the picture. Each team should also appoint an observer to use the communication and team roles checklists.

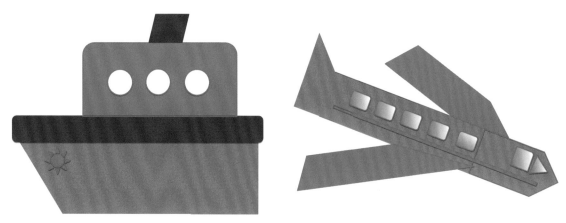

Figure 5.2 Examples of pictures for ice-breaker activity 2

The observer

The observer will not draw a picture, but will observe both the 'describer' and the 'drawers' throughout the task, and will report back at the end using the teamwork checklists.

The activity

The nominated describer should be given 1 minute to study the allocated picture.

The describer will communicate to the rest of the team the exact content of the picture that is in front of them, abiding by the rules at all times. The rules are presented on PowerPoint slides entitled *PROMPT ice-breaker activities* (see box).

At the end of the activity

Stop the activity after 3 minutes. At the end of the activity, all the drawings can be attached to the wall for each team to compare. The team is then shown the original picture.

Rules of ice-breaker activity 2: draw a picture

1. **Nouns** (naming words) that identify the object(s) to be drawn *must not* be used, e.g.

   ▪ name of object: e.g. cow, tractor, tree, sky, field

   ▪ type of object: e.g. vehicle, animal, vegetation

2. **Adjectives** (describing words) *can* be used: e.g. large, small, circular.

3. **Verbs** (doing words) *can* be used: e.g. 'draw a circle in the middle of the paper'.

4. Hands and body language *must not* be used: i.e. no facial expressions or eye movements to suggest an idea, or use of hands.

5. The only question that *can* be asked is: 'Can you repeat that, please?'

   ▪ **The describer will have 3 minutes to describe what is in front of them.**

   ▪ **The participants should not be able to look at other group members' drawings.**

   ▪ **The participants must draw only what they are told to draw.**

After the activity

There are usually quite surprising results at the end!

Feedback

Trainers should facilitate the discussion all together:

■ First, each describer should comment on how easy they thought it was to communicate with their team.

■ Then the drawers should comment on how easy it was to understand the instructions they were given.

■ Finally, the observers should give feedback using the communication and team roles checklists.

The team that produces the pictures that are most like the original may be given a prize!

Ice-breaker activity 2: draw a picture – teamwork checklists

Communication		YES	NO
State the problem	Clinical problem was stated clearly to arriving team		
Instructions	Instructions were clearly worded		
	Unnecessary conversation/noise was avoided		
	Action plans were shared		
	Goals were clearly identified		
Addressed	Specific instructions were given to the appropriate team members		
Sent	Communication was not rushed		
	It was clear what action was required		
Heard	Acknowledgements were made		
	Requests for repeat information were made		
Understood	The information was understood and repeated back by recipient		
	The correct action was performed		

Team roles and leadership		YES	NO
Roles	Each team member had a clear role		
	There was a team leader		
Adaptability	Team members responded well to different situations		
Responsibility	Team members assumed responsibility for their role		
Advocate	Tasks were delegated appropriately		
Feedback	There were regular updates on progress		
	A running commentary was provided		
Support	Team members did not argue about issues		
	None of the team members decided to 'go it alone'		

Section 6
Basic life support and maternal collapse

Key learning points

- To recognise maternal collapse and call for the clinical emergency team/cardiac arrest team (2222) early for clinical emergencies, peri-arrest and/or cardiac arrest.
- Cardiac disease is the commonest cause of maternal death in the UK.
- Recognition, assessment and resuscitation of maternal collapse:
  - ☐ A B C approach
  - ☐ Manual left uterine displacement (or 15–30° left tilt if on firm tilting surface, e.g. operating table) to reduce aortocaval compression
  - ☐ Use of an automated external defibrillator (AED) if available
- Calling for help: effective communication of the problem to the team.
- Equipment: knowing where to find emergency trolley, defibrillator, anaphylaxis box.
- Appropriate documentation.

Common difficulties observed in training drills

- Failure to call for senior help in a deteriorating pregnant/postnatal woman
- Not starting basic life support
- Forgetting to keep woman supine with manual left uterine displacement during cardiopulmonary resuscitation (CPR)
- Not administering high-flow oxygen to mother
- Not using an AED to assess rhythm and defibrillate, if needed

Aims of the basic life support scenario

This scenario allows midwives, obstetricians, anaesthetists, healthcare support workers, and student midwives and doctors to gain experience of performing basic life support in a pregnant woman. Emphasis is placed on teaching staff to recognise this rare problem and to work as a team to resuscitate the mother.

Supporting material

The downloadable supporting materials included are:

- Basic life support algorithm
- Blank maternity notes

These are all in a printable format and for use in the scenario.

Basic life support scenario

This case presents a 37-year-old woman in her first pregnancy. She is attending her community antenatal clinic for a routine appointment at 32 weeks. She is reviewed by the midwife and complains that she has been feeling increasingly short of breath over the last few days. She suddenly collapses, becomes cyanosed and gasps for breath, and then proceeds to have a cardiac arrest. The multi-professional team is required to recognise the maternal cardiac arrest, call for appropriate help and commence immediate basic life support.

> You are running an antenatal clinic at a GP surgery. A woman in her first pregnancy has attended for her routine appointment at 32 weeks. She tells you that she has been feeling short of breath over the last few days. She suddenly collapses, turns blue and starts gasping for breath.

Equipment

- Basic life support mannequins (e.g. Resusci-Anne): one mannequin per team
- AED training defibrillator or cardboard-box AED (see **Appendix 3**)
- Guedel airway

- Bag/valve mask
- Cushion or 'magic pants' to simulate pregnant uterus

Instructions for drill facilitators

- Involve your hospital's resuscitation training department and/or an obstetric anaesthetist for the training of basic and advanced life support.
- Divide the participants into small groups around each mannequin.
- Set the scene using the scenario provided.
- Ask the participants to perform basic life support manoeuvres in pairs.
- Encourage all the participants to 'have a go'.

Use the basic life support algorithm to prompt and guide where needed (Figure 6.1).

Debrief and feedback

The importance of early detection of the deteriorating woman before cardiac arrest occurs cannot be overemphasised. However, this scenario presents with an unexpected cardiac arrest in the GP surgery.

Explain to the participants that there is evidence that relying on a check of the carotid pulse to diagnose cardiac arrest is unreliable and time-consuming; checking for breathing is also prone to error (as agonal gasps are often misdiagnosed as normal breathing). Therefore, the 2015 Resuscitation Council guidelines stress that *the absence of normal breathing continues to be the main sign of cardiac arrest in a non-responsive victim*.[1] If a person is breathing abnormally and shows no signs of life, then basic life support must be commenced immediately.

Cardiopulmonary resuscitation (CPR) should be stopped only if the woman shows signs of regaining consciousness (e.g. coughing, opening her eyes, speaking or moving purposefully), or breathing normally.

Explain that if you are on your own you should use your mobile phone to call for help. Only leave the woman (and stop CPR) if there is no other way of getting help.

If help is available, they should be asked to dial 999 for an ambulance (or if in hospital dial 2222 for the maternal cardiac arrest team) and bring

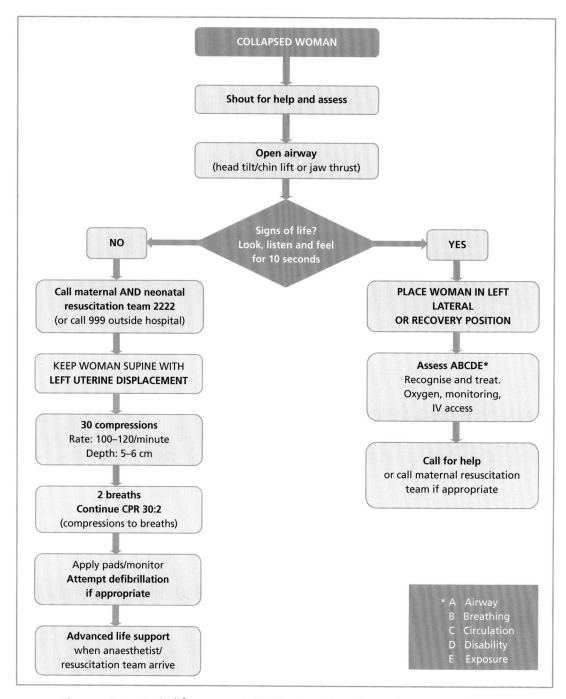

Figure 6.1 Basic life support (BLS) algorithm (based on Resuscitation Council (UK) Guidelines, 2015)

an automated external defibrillator (AED), if available. Stress that chest compressions should be started immediately. Compressions should be applied to the centre of the sternum at a rate of 100–120 compressions per minute and to a depth of 5–6 cm.

After 30 compressions, two breaths should be given (using a bag and mask or Laerdel pocket mask, if available – or consider mouth to mouth if outside hospital with no equipment).

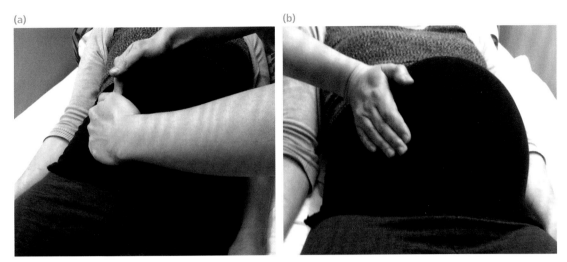

Figure 6.2 Manual displacement of the uterus to the left in a collapsed pregnant woman: (a) from the mother's left side, pulling the uterus with two hands, or (b) from the mother's right side, using one hand to push the uterus

Chest compressions and rescue breaths should be continued in a ratio of 30:2 for as long as necessary, with team members swapping over as they get tired.

Explain the importance of minimising the interruptions to chest compressions, as rescue breaths, rhythm checks and checking for signs of life should take no more than 5 seconds and should be immediately followed by a further 30 chest compressions.

Stress that aortocaval compression should be kept to a minimum, and that the resuscitator can administer more effective cardiac compressions if the woman is supine. Therefore, the woman should be kept supine, with her uterus manually displaced to the left to reduce aortocaval compression (Figure 6.2), unless she is on a firm tilting surface (e.g. operating table), when the 15–30° left tilt position can be used.

Explain how the use of an AED is now recommended as part of basic life support; if you have a training defibrillator, then this too could be used during the scenario. Also, emphasise the importance of commencing advanced life support and performing perimortem caesarean section or operative vaginal birth as soon as possible (in less than 5 minutes if resuscitation is unsuccessful) and that the team in the hospital would need to be prepared for this on arrival. Discussions should also include stressing that if arrest occurs outside of the hospital, it is imperative to continue good basic life support and left manual displacement to keep the woman's vital organs oxygenated throughout transfer in the ambulance. In addition, since perimortem birth gives the best chance of saving the life of the mother (and the baby), emphasise the urgency of moving the woman to hospital and avoiding prolonged resuscitation attempts on the scene.[2]

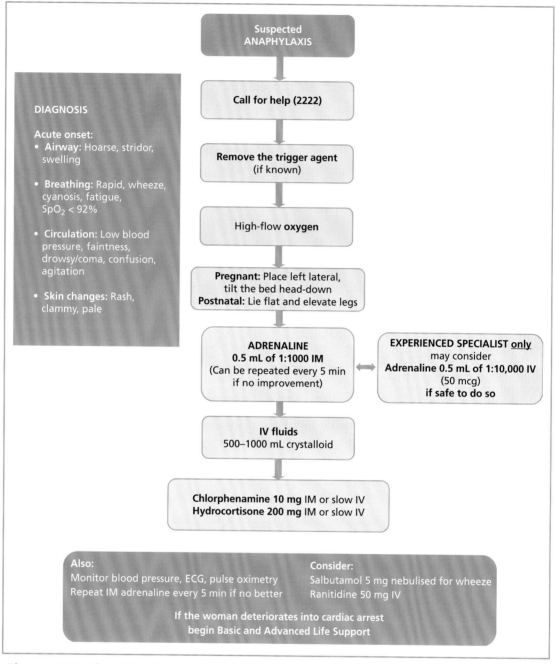

Figure 6.3 Algorithm for the management of anaphylaxis (based on Resuscitation Council (UK) Guidelines 2015)

Anaphylaxis scenario

This BLS scenario could be combined with an anaphylactic reaction to a medicine or allergen. One circumstance that may occur on the labour ward is an anaphylactic reaction to an intravenous iron infusion. The scenario would require the team to perform BLS and left manual displacement, but

Location of anaphylaxis boxes on labour ward

1. **Resuscitation trolley:** labour ward theatre corridor

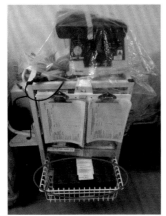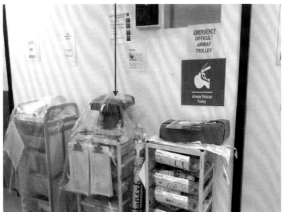

2. **Labour ward recovery area:** in blue emergency drug box on
   end shelf in theatre recovery (by the window)

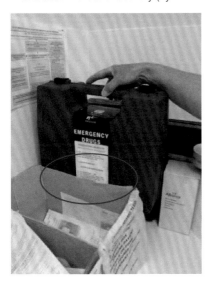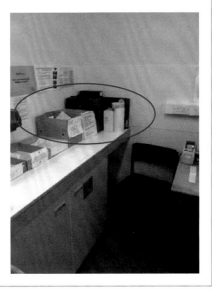

Figure 6.4 Example of information sheet for location of emergency
medications box

also administer adrenaline (epinephrine) and IV fluids as per the anaphylaxis algorithm (Figure 6.3). It is also an important scenario to ensure that all maternity staff know the location of the emergency medications box within your clinical areas. It may be helpful to take photographs of the location of these boxes and add this information into your local pre-reading booklet (Figure 6.4).

Basic life support scenario: clinical checklist

		Time	✓
Responsiveness	Shake and shout		
	Open airway and check for normal breathing for up to 10 seconds by looking, listening and feeling		
Call for help	Use bystander or mobile phone		
	Call 999 (or 2222 in hospital) and state 'maternal cardiac arrest' (include neonatal team)		
	Ask for automated external defibrillator (AED)		
Compressions	Immediately start chest compressions		
	Rate 100–120 per minute		
	Centre of chest		
	Depth 5–6 cm		
	Minimal breaks		
	Ratio 30 compressions to 2 breaths		
Ventilations	2 breaths (1 second each)		
	Using bag and mask (or mouth to mouth if outside hospital and no equipment available)		
	Observe for chest movement		
Displacement	Keep woman supine and manually displace uterus to the left, or tilt if on firm tilting surface		
Defibrillation	Attempt defibrillation with training AED		
Advanced life support	Commence ALS as soon as possible		
Documentation	Timings of events		
	Actions performed		
	Persons present		

References

1. Resuscitation Council (UK). *Resuscitation Guidelines* 2015. www.resus.org.uk (accessed August 2017).

2. Knight M, Nair M, Tuffnell D, *et al.* (eds.); MBRRACE-UK. *Saving Lives, Improving Mothers' Care: Surveillance of Maternal Deaths in the UK 2012–14 and Lessons Learned to Inform Maternity Care from the UK and Ireland Confidential Enquiries into Maternal Deaths and Morbidity 2009–14*. Oxford: National Perinatal Epidemiology Unit, University of Oxford, 2016.

Section 7

Maternal cardiac arrest and advanced life support

Key learning points

- Recall the causes of maternal cardiac arrest.
- Management of maternal cardiac arrest using advanced life support (ALS) algorithm.
- The importance of left manual uterine displacement to reduce aortocaval compression after 20 weeks gestation.
- Perform perimortem caesarean (or operative vaginal birth) immediately if resuscitation is unsuccessful.
- Document details of management accurately, clearly and legibly.

Common difficulties observed in training drills

- Failing to recognise cardiac arrest and therefore not starting life support in a timely manner
- Concentrating on ALS and neglecting to perform good-quality basic life support (BLS)
- Not manually displacing the uterus
- Not connecting the defibrillator
- Unnecessary interruption of cardiac compressions
- Failure to understand that perimortem caesarean section is primarily performed for maternal resuscitation

■ Moving the woman to the operating theatre to perform the perimortem caesarean section

■ Delaying the commencement of perimortem caesarean section

■ Forgetting to call the neonatal team

Aims of the advanced life support scenario

In this scenario, the team should recognise cardiac arrest, call for appropriate help (including the maternal cardiac arrest team), immediately commence basic life support, and commence ALS as soon as possible.

Supporting material

The downloadable supporting materials included are:

■ Treatment algorithms for basic and advanced life support

■ Maternity notes

■ Examples of ECG strips: sinus rhythm, ventricular tachycardia, ventricular fibrillation, asystole

■ Pictures of a perimortem caesarean section set and automated external defibrillator (AED).

These are all in a printable format for use in the scenario.

Advanced life support scenario

A woman runs into the antenatal ward office to tell staff that her pregnant sister has collapsed and she thinks she has stopped breathing. The scenario enables staff and students to practise basic and advanced life support for a pregnant woman.

This scenario is a maternal cardiac arrest on the antenatal ward with a suspected amniotic fluid embolism. An additional scenario that covers advanced life support is presented in Section 8 (anaesthetic emergencies), relating to the management of local anaesthetic toxicity.

The first handover is given to two members of staff in the antenatal ward office by one drill facilitator (playing the handing-over midwife). At the end of this handover, a second drill facilitator (playing Helen's sister) runs into the room announcing that her sister has collapsed. On arrival in the ward area, Helen is found lying on the floor and has no signs of life.

Drill facilitator 1 (handing over to the midwife)

'Helen has been admitted for induction of labour. She is 40+12 weeks of gestation in her first pregnancy. She was given a Propess pessary 4 hours ago and has been contracting strongly for the past hour. Helen's now wanting some stronger pain relief and so needs to be transferred up to the labour ward. I would be grateful if you could transfer Helen up there for me.'

Drill facilitator 2 (Helen's sister)

'Help, help! My sister's waters have just broken and she suddenly complained that she was feeling unwell and then collapsed on the floor. I don't think she is breathing. Come quickly, please help her.'

Equipment

- Full-body mannequin, e.g. SimMom (Laerdal, Norway) or a basic resuscitation half-mannequin such as Resusci-Anne
- Pregnant uterus and fetus (use 'magic pants' – large pair of pants with a Velcro incision, cushion and a baby doll) if using a basic mannequin – see **Appendix 3**
- Skin with caesarean section incision and fetus if using a SimMom mannequin or a PROMPT Flex with caesarean section skin as the bottom half of the Resuci-Anne half-mannequin
- Wig, bra and clothes to make mannequin more realistic
- Cardiac arrest trolley (training trolley and drugs if possible):
  - ☐ Guedel airway
  - ☐ bag and mask
  - ☐ intubation equipment
  - ☐ drugs: 1 mg of adrenaline (epinephrine) – use 10 mL syringes labelled adrenaline (epinephrine)
  - ☐ IV cannulae with needles removed
  - ☐ IV crystalloid and giving sets

☐ blood bottles and forms

☐ stethoscope

- Perimortem caesarean section kit (or photograph)
- Defibrillator and pads

  ☐ training AED (if available), programmed to not require a shock

  ☐ or a cardboard-box defibrillator (see **Appendix 3**)

- Laminated ECG cardiac arrest rhythms: VF, VT, sinus, asystole

- Doppler and CTG machine or laminated pictures (you would not expect these to be used during the scenario, but they can be available in case participants ask for them)
- Maternity notes
- Laminated clinical and teamwork checklists, with pens

Setting-up instructions

It is a good idea to involve your hospital's resuscitation training department in the planning of an ALS drill; if possible, the resuscitation officer may facilitate the scenario along with the obstetric anaesthetist and a midwife.

- Make sure the mannequin is dressed and has a pregnant abdomen containing a baby with skin that can be 'incised' to perform a perimortem caesarean section (or Velcro that can be opened).
- Place the mannequin on the floor in a room near some chairs, as if she has collapsed off the chair and slipped to the floor.
- Prepare a training cardiac arrest trolley containing the equipment outlined above. Clearly label this 'TRAINING CARDIAC ARREST TROLLEY' and if possible place this near the real cardiac arrest trolley, so that participants learn where the actual trolley is kept. If you are carrying out the training away from the clinical area, have the trolley nearby, outside the room.
- If you are using a training AED, ensure that you have programmed it to recognise a non-shockable rhythm when it is attached to the patient.
- Ensure that the maternity notes have been printed off and are near the woman.

Instructions for drill facilitators

The first facilitator should start the handover to two members of the team outside the ward area (the rest of the team should be waiting in an appropriate separate area). As this handover is finishing, the second facilitator should run out of the room where the mannequin is situated and announce that Helen has collapsed.

If there is a team observing the drill, they should stand in the corner of the ward area to observe the scenario, and two of the team can be allocated the task of ticking off the clinical and teamwork checklists.

Following the handover, the facilitator should also stand in the corner of the room. If there is no other team observing, one of the facilitators should complete the clinical and teamwork checklists.

As specific team members are requested to help, the facilitator should go to the door and ask them to attend the emergency. If the emergency buzzer is used, all the team members should be asked to attend. When the team check for signs of life, say: 'There are no signs of life.'

Participants should follow the algorithm for the management of maternal cardiac arrest (Figure 7.1). If you are not using a pre-programmed training AED (but your unit uses an AED), say 'no shock advised.'

The team is expected to immediately call for additional help using the emergency bell, check for signs of life by 'shaking and shouting', and open the airway to 'look, listen and feel' for breathing for up to 10 seconds. In this scenario there are no signs of life.

At this point one team member should go to get help, make sure the arrest trolley containing the defibrillator is on its way, and ensure that a 2222 emergency call has been made to the switchboard announcing 'maternal cardiac arrest'. While help is being summoned, the second team member should immediately commence 30 chest compressions followed by two rescue breaths.

When help arrives, they should displace Helen's uterus so it does not compress the inferior vena cava by asking an assistant to manually move her uterus to the left.

Someone should make a note of the time that the arrest occurred and request that the team prepare for a perimortem caesarean section.

The additional staff should help with ventilation. If an anaesthetist has not yet arrived, the team should use a Guedel airway and a 'bag and mask' or a Laerdal pocket mask to provide ventilations at a ratio of 30 compressions to

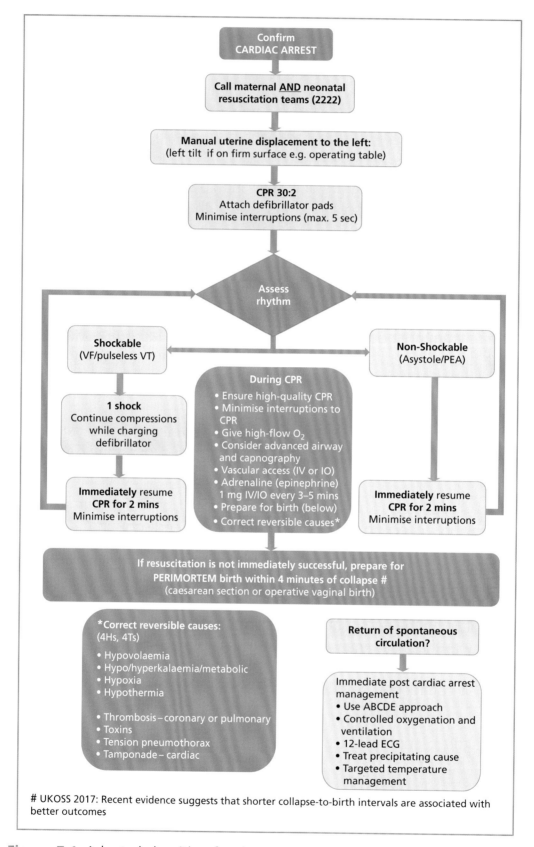

Figure 7.1 Adapted algorithm for the management of maternal cardiac arrest

2 breaths. Once an anaesthetist has arrived, they should secure a definitive airway with an endotracheal tube. Once the airway is secured with an endotracheal tube, continual chest compressions should be performed to a depth of 5–6 cm (at a rate of 100–120 per minute), with simultaneous ventilations (at a rate of approximately 12 per minute).

The defibrillator should be attached to the woman as soon as possible and, if required, a shock given. The team should be aware of their own safety when using the defibrillator. In this scenario there is no shockable rhythm; the woman has pulseless electrical activity (PEA) and therefore defibrillation is not required. (The local anaesthetic toxicity scenario presented in **Section 8b** contains a shockable rhythm requiring defibrillation.)

The urgent birth of the baby should be undertaken as soon as possible after the arrest if there has been no recovery of the maternal circulation, and definitely within 5 minutes of effective CPR; the team should immediately make plans to achieve this. Birth in this case will require a perimortem caesarean section, as Helen is still in early labour.

Helen will develop signs of life after the baby has been born. At this point you can stop the scenario.

> **It is important that the team is sufficiently supported by the facilitators so that Helen survives, making it a positive experience for the participants.**

Prompts

Here are some suggestions to prompt the team if they are struggling with the scenario:

If collapse is not noted:	'Why isn't she talking to me?'
	'Do something, she isn't breathing!'
If help is not called:	'Where are the doctors?'
If CPR is not commenced:	'Why aren't you doing anything for her?'
If the situation is not explained to her, Helen's sister can become distressed, agitated, pacing around and asking questions about the resuscitation.	
If a perimortem caesarean section is not considered:	'What about the baby?'

Debrief and feedback

In the debrief at the end of the scenario, remind participants that maternal cardiac arrest in the UK is extremely uncommon, and most maternity staff will not have encountered this situation. Maternal cardiac arrest is an extremely stressful situation for everyone involved and needs to be managed as efficiently as possible.

The importance of immediately starting cardiac chest compressions cannot be overstated. Staff are often reluctant to commence CPR in case the woman has not really collapsed. If there are no signs of life (look, listen and feel for normal breath sounds for up to 10 seconds) then 30 chest compressions must be started as soon as 2222/999 has been called. Discuss the fact that agonal breathing is not normal and that CPR is required in this situation.

In addition, stress the importance of only stopping cardiac compressions for key events (e.g. to give ventilation breaths until a secure airway has been achieved, or during defibrillation). Compressions should not be stopped for any other reason (e.g. when help arrives, to attach the defibrillator pads, while charging the defibrillator or during birth of the baby). Chest compressions are essential to keep oxygenated blood circulating to the woman's vital organs. Without effective chest compressions, the woman will not survive.

Remember to demonstrate how to perform manual displacement of the uterus (assistant kneeling/standing on the mother's left side and pulling the uterus towards her with two hands, or assistant kneeling/standing on the mother's right side and using one hand to push her uterus towards her left (see Figure 6.2). Effective cardiac compressions require the chest to be supine; therefore, discuss how manual left uterine displacement is preferable unless the woman is on a hard surface such as an operating table, when left tilt can be used.

Discuss how the fetus is delivered in order to improve the chances of maternal survival. If the uterine size measures above the umbilicus and the woman has not recovered with CPR, then the baby's birth should be expedited: traditionally we have aimed to do this within 5 minutes, but birth should not be delayed once CPR has been unsuccessful, as even shorter collapse-to-birth intervals are associated with better outcomes.[1]

Birth of the baby improves maternal survival because:

- The baby is no longer 'stealing' oxygen from the mother.
- The fetoplacental unit is no longer diverting the maternal circulating volume.
- The uterus is no longer pressing on the inferior vena cava, preventing venous return to the heart.

Ventilation will be easier without a large uterus pressing up on the diaphragm. All these factors make resuscitation with an empty uterus much more effective.

In almost every case of maternal cardiac arrest, a perimortem caesarean section will be required to facilitate the birth of the baby. However, if the woman is in the second stage of labour and the baby is low in the pelvis, an operative vaginal birth with forceps may be performed (as in the scenario presented in Section 8b).

Whenever possible, the perimortem caesarean section or operative vaginal birth should be performed in the location where the maternal cardiac arrest has occurred, as moving the woman to theatre at such a crucial stage will compromise the effectiveness of CPR and cause delay. Staff should be reminded to make their working area as unrestricted as possible – in this scenario, by moving the chairs out of the way, but in other scenarios by moving the bed into the middle of the room and removing the end of the bed.

While a perimortem birth is performed for resuscitation of the mother and not to save the baby, the baby may well be born alive, and the team should make sure that the neonatal team is in attendance and is prepared for a concurrent neonatal resuscitation.

Explain to the participants that most causes of maternal cardiac arrest (e.g. pulmonary embolism, haemorrhage, amniotic fluid embolism) do not result in a shockable rhythm, and therefore defibrillation is unlikely to be necessary. However, the defibrillator should be attached as soon as possible and, if required, a shock should be immediately administered. All staff should be familiar with the location and workings of the defibrillator in their unit. Staff should also know where they can easily locate a perimortem caesarean section pack if a woman collapses. If your unit does not already have a perimortem caesarean section set, you may wish to think about placing a set (with a disposable scalpel) in every antenatal area. Figure 7.2 shows the contents of a perimorten caesarean pack.

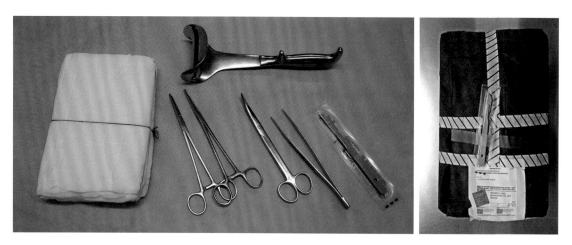

Figure 7.2 Suggested contents of a perimortem caesarean pack

- Sterile disposable scalpel (attached to outside of pack to maintain sterility of pack contents)
- 1 pack of large taped swabs
- 1 Doyen's retractor
- 2–3 clamps (Kocher's, Spencer Wells or similar)
- 1 large dissecting scissors (e.g. Mayo scissors)
- 1 toothed dissecting forceps
- Also: gloves ± gown for the operator (can be outside the pack)

References

1. Beckett VA, Knight M, Sharpe P. The CAPS Study: incidence, management and outcomes of cardiac arrest in pregnancy in the UK: a prospective, descriptive study. *BJOG* 2017; 124: 1374–81.

Maternal cardiac arrest scenario: clinical checklist

		Time	✓
Call for help	Activate emergency bell		
	Call 2222 and state 'maternal cardiac arrest' and location of incident		
	Call neonatal cardiac arrest team		
Equipment	Ask for cardiac arrest trolley, perimortem caesarean section pack and resuscitaire		
Position of mother	Manual left uterine displacement		
Assess	Check own safety to approach		
	Check responsiveness, colour, movement		
Airway	Check airway		
	Open/protect airway		
Breathing (look, listen, feel)	Check breathing looking for movement of chest, listen for breath sounds, feel for air on cheek (for up to 10 seconds)		
	If not breathing, start chest compressions		
Circulation	Chest compressions – 30 compressions to 2 breaths, rate 100–120 per minute. Depth 5–6 cm		
	Attach defibrillator/monitor and assess rhythm		
	Assess rhythm – shockable or non-shockable		
	Continue chest compressions while defibrillator charging		
IV access	Insert large-bore IV cannula and take bloods		
Medication	1 mg adrenaline (epinephrine) IV every 3–5 minutes		
Prepare for perimortem birth	If resuscitation unsuccessful, prepare for perimortem birth within 5 minutes of collapse		
Documentation	Time of arrest		
	Arrival time and persons present		
	Timings of defibrillation, drugs administered, time of birth of baby and time cardiac output regained		

Maternal cardiac arrest scenario: teamwork checklists

Communication		YES	NO
State the problem	Clinical problem was stated clearly to arriving team		
Instructions	Instructions were clearly worded		
	Unnecessary conversation/noise was avoided		
	Action plans were shared		
	Goals were clearly identified		
Addressed	Specific instructions were given to the appropriate team members		
Sent	Communication was not rushed		
	It was clear what action was required		
Heard	Acknowledgements were made		
	Requests for repeat information were made		
Understood	The information was understood and repeated back by recipient		
	The correct action was performed		

Team roles and leadership		YES	NO
Roles	Each team member had a clear role		
	There was a team leader		
Adaptability	Team members responded well to different situations		
Responsibility	Team members assumed responsibility for their role		
Advocate	Tasks were delegated appropriately		
Feedback	There were regular updates on progress		
	A running commentary was provided		
Support	Team members did not argue about issues		
	None of the team members decided to 'go it alone'		

Section 8
Maternal anaesthetic emergencies

Key learning points

- To understand the difficulties of intubating the obstetric patient.
- To understand team roles in the management of failed intubation.
- To understand the role of intrauterine fetal resuscitation in potentially avoiding the need for general anaesthesia.
- Recognition and management of high regional block.
- Signs and symptoms of local anaesthetic toxicity.
- Management of cardiac arrest in a patient with local anaesthetic toxicity.

Introduction

We have included three different scenarios in this section which are relevant to the key anaesthetic emergencies explained in Module 4 of the *Course Manual*. The scenarios are:

- 8a: Failed tracheal intubation
- 8b: Local anaesthetic toxicity
- 8c: Total spinal block

There are also specific key learning points incorporated at the start of each emergency scenario.

Section 8a: Failed tracheal intubation

Key learning points

- The importance of good preparation: woman, equipment, position, pre-oxygenation.
- Effective communication with theatre and obstetric team.
- Prioritise oxygenation over intubation.
- Declare emergency and call for help.
- Follow failed tracheal intubation algorithm.

Common difficulties observed in training drills

- Unfamiliarity with own equipment
- Failure to declare emergency
- Persisting with intubation attempts
- Not calling for senior help

Aims of the failed intubation scenario

The aim of this scenario is for all members of the maternity team to participate in a failed intubation drill, ideally in the surroundings of their own labour ward theatres. This allows the anaesthetic team to familiarise themselves with their local difficult intubation equipment and where to find it. It also gives the opportunity to practise the communication required between the anaesthetic and maternity teams; and the maternity staff will gain an understanding of their supportive role in this emergency situation.

Supporting material

The downloadable supporting materials included are:

- Treatment algorithm for failed intubation (based on Obstetric Anaesthetists' Association (OAA)/Difficult Airway Society (DAS) Obstetric Airway Guidelines 2015)[1]

- The OAA-DAS 2015 decision-making tool
- Maternity notes
- Failed intubation scenario checklists

These are all in a printable format for use in the scenario.

Failed intubation scenario

This scenario presents a woman in her first pregnancy requiring a general anaesthetic for a category 1 caesarean section who is found to be difficult to intubate. The scenario enables anaesthetists, theatre staff, obstetricians, midwives and healthcare support workers to gain experience of the immediate management and team working required during a difficult intubation. The team are required to support and assist the anaesthetist in managing this rare and very acute emergency. Management should include calling for senior help and following the failed intubation algorithm so that the mother's respirations are restored and the maternity team can continue to assist the birth of the baby.

'Sarah is a 30-year-old woman in her first pregnancy. She is in early labour at 40 weeks' gestation and requires a category 1 caesarean section (CS) for a pathological cardiotocograph trace (it was impossible to carry out fetal blood sampling (FBS) at this early stage of labour).

She is an asthmatic with a booking body mass index (BMI) of 38. She has no allergies. She has had a previous general anaesthetic (GA) aged 25 for appendicitis and this was uneventful.

Sarah is very anxious and refusing a spinal anaesthetic. She is in theatre, where the anaesthetic machine, equipment and drugs have been checked. The anaesthetic assistant is fully trained, but might not be known to the anaesthetist. The obstetrician performing the CS and the midwife looking after Sarah are in theatre with her.'

Equipment

- Mannequin such as SimMom (Laerdal, Norway), ideally intubatable and set up for failed intubation; or a basic resuscitation mannequin such as a Resusci-Anne

☐ SimMom: place fetus/baby doll in pelvis, and apply the caesarean section skin

☐ Other mannequin (Resusci-Anne): place fetus/baby doll into caesarean section 'magic pants'

☐ Wig, bra and patient gown

■ Obstetric intubation trolley or difficult intubation equipment as available in your unit, e.g. including McCoy blade laryngoscope, smaller tube sizes, first- and second-generation supraglottic devices such as laryngeal mask airway (LMA), i-gel, Proseal LMA; front-of-neck equipment, e.g. scalpel, tracheal hook/dilator, size 6.0 endotracheal tube

■ Pillow under head of mannequin

■ Anaesthetic assistant (either a proper anaesthetic assistant, who is a participant on the course, or faculty acting as an anaesthetic assistant)

■ Anaesthetic machine set up and prepared as for caesarean section (CS) under general anaesthesia (GA)

■ ECG leads, NIBP, capnography and SpO_2 monitor

■ Laptop with software to generate the clinical signs for the monitor (e.g. Laerdal simulation software); or a tablet to use as a monitor, running simulation software (e.g. SimMon application, Castle Anderson); or laminated monitor readings

■ Caesarean section set (reduced set of non-sterile instruments)

■ Needleless intravenous cannulae

■ Intravenous crystalloid

■ 1–2 × 20 mL syringe labelled as thiopental/propofol as used on your unit

■ 2 × 2 mL syringes labelled suxamethonium, or 5–10 mL syringe labelled rocuronium

■ Anaesthetic chart

■ Laminated failed intubation algorithm

■ Laminated OAA-DAS 2015 decision-making tool

■ Laminated failed intubation clinical and teamwork checklists and pens

NOTE: If you are unable to utilise all the real equipment and run the scenario in your operating theatre, you may need to use sets of laminated photographs showing an anaesthetic machine, monitoring and appropriate failed intubation equipment.

Setting-up instructions

Ideally you will be able to run this scenario in your obstetric theatre with your own obstetric anaesthetic intubation trolley (Figure 8a.1). If not, the scenario can still be run with different or more limited equipment (see equipment list above). If you do not want the team to know what the emergency is going to be, then you may call this the 'category 1 caesarean section' drill.

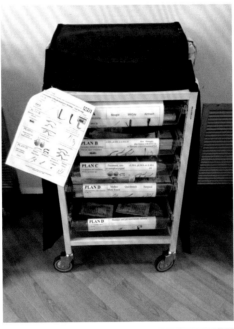

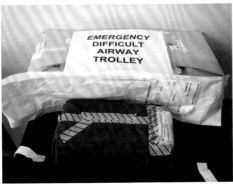

Figure 8a.1 Example of difficult intubation trolley (based on Difficult Airway Society (DAS) guidelines)

The obstetrician, midwife and HCA/MCA participants should assume their usual roles during this category 1 CS. The anaesthetic assistant can either be an anaesthetic assistant who is a participant on the course, or an anaesthetist who is a participant. Alternatively, one of the anaesthetic faculty could be the anaesthetic assistant.

Depending on the complexity of the mannequin and the scenario, set it up as unintubatable and/or unventilatable. If only a normal resuscitation mannequin is available, the drill instructor will have to direct the participant as to whether they are able to get a view of the larynx, or able/unable to intubate or ventilate. If you are able to run this scenario in an operating theatre, place the mannequin on the operating table with monitoring (as described above) attached and the table on a left tilt.

Pre-induction preparation, communication with the anaesthetic assistant and effective pre-oxygenation are other key points to be covered in the scenario. The drill can also be adjusted to practise both 'can't intubate but *can* ventilate' and 'can't intubate and *can't* ventilate' situations.

Instructions for drill facilitators

This drill should be led by an experienced anaesthetist.

Hand over Sarah's history and reasons for needing a category 1 CS under GA. Give full details such that the anaesthetist taking handover can start pre-oxygenation almost immediately. The CTG should be discontinued and the obstetrician should begin surgical preparation of the abdomen.

Once thiopental/propofol and suxamethonium/rocuronium are given allow the anaesthetist from the participating team to attempt intubation. Set the mannequin to be unintubatable or if using a Resusci-Anne, the drill facilitator should control the scenario with clear instructions that the mannequin is unintubatable. The participating anaesthetist should declare the emergency i.e. 'we have a failed intubation', so that the surgeon, theatre staff and midwife cease preparations for the operative procedure.

Thereafter, control the scenario as required to evolve along an unventilatable path until the participant chooses a specific adjunct. Depending on the situation, the oxygen saturations should fall steadily until ventilation is restored.

Encourage the participants to call for help early and follow the failed intubation algorithm (use local guideline or example in Figure 8a.2). Should

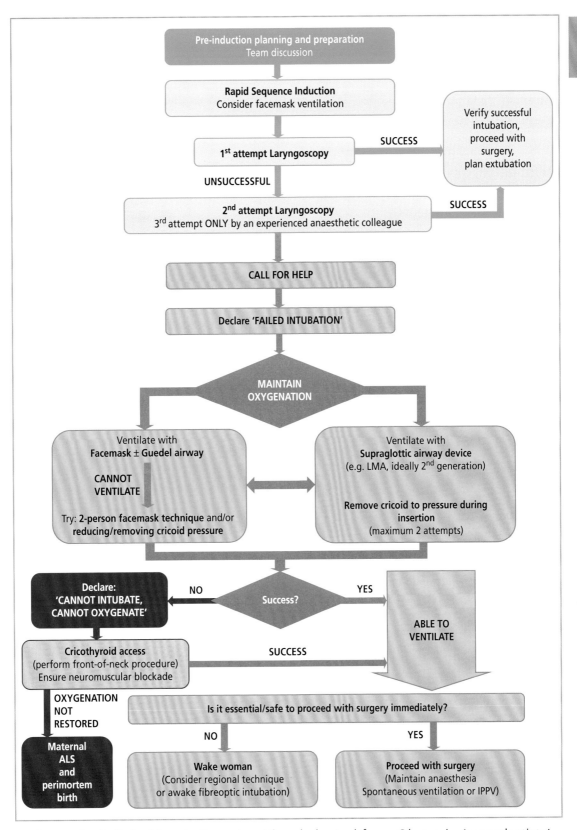

Figure 8a.2 Failed intubation algorithm (adapted from Obstetric Anaesthetists' Association/Difficult Airway Society)

the mannequin arrest, the team should move on to the maternal cardiac arrest drill and perimortem CS.

The scenario should end with restoration of ventilation. If possible, once the debrief is completed, aim to repeat the scenario allowing another anaesthetist to be the main participant.

> **It is important that the team are supported by the facilitators sufficiently so that Sarah survives, making it a positive experience for the participants.**

Prompts

Below are some suggestions to prompt the team if they are struggling with the scenario:

If there are repeated attempts at intubation:	'The oxygen saturations are falling'
If the anaesthetist continues with repeated attempts:	'Would you like to stop attempts at intubation and call for senior help?'
If they fail to declare emergency:	Ask if they would like to 'Declare the emergency'
If they fail to call for help:	'Would you like to call for help?'
If they are unsure what to do:	Support and guide them using the failed intubation algorithm

Debrief and feedback

Ideally the scenario is run with the multi-professional team, so that communication between all members of the team is encouraged. Use the clinical and communication checklists to aid the debrief.

Include discussions regarding the problems with general anaesthesia in the pregnant woman and also when it might be appropriate to continue with the CS without intubation. The OAA-DAS 2015 decision-making tool may be used in support (Figure 8a.3).

Ideas for roles and responsibilities of all team members in this situation may be highlighted. This should include how, in this situation, the anaesthetist would lead the emergency and ensure that the surgeon does not continue with the operative procedure until the anaesthetist is happy that adequate ventilation is restored.

Table 1– proceed with surgery?				
Factors to consider	**WAKE**	◄──────────────────►		**PROCEED**
Before induction / Maternal condition	• No compromise	• Mild acute compromise	• Haemorrhage responsive to resuscitation	• Hypovolaemia requiring corrective surgery • Critical cardiac or respiratory compromise, cardiac arrest
Fetal condition	• No compromise	• Compromise corrected with intrauterine resuscitation, pH < 7.2 but > 7.15	• Continuing fetal heart rate abnormality despite intrauterine resuscitation, pH < 7.15	• Sustained bradycardia • Fetal haemorrhage • Suspected uterine rupture
Anaesthetist	• Novice	• Junior trainee	• Senior trainee	• Consultant / specialist
Obesity	• Supermorbid	• Morbid	• Obese	• Normal
Surgical factors	• Complex surgery or major haemorrhage anticipated	• Multiple uterine scars • Some surgical difficulties expected	• Single uterine scar	• No risk factors
Aspiration risk	• Recent food	• No recent food • In labour • Opioids given • Antacids not given	• No recent food • In labour • Opioids not given • Antacids not given	• Fasted • Not in labour • Antacids given
Alternative anaesthesia • regional • securing airway awake	• No anticipated difficulty	• Predicted difficulty	• Relatively contraindicated	• Absolutely contraindicated or has failed • Surgery started
After failed intubation / Airway device / ventilation	• Difficult facemask ventilation • Front-of-neck	• Adequate facemask ventilation	• First generation supraglottic airway device	• Second generation supraglottic airway device
Airway hazards	• Laryngeal oedema • Stridor	• Bleeding • Trauma	• Secretions	• None evident

Criteria to be used in the decision to wake or proceed following failed tracheal intubation. In any individual patient, some factors may suggest waking and others proceeding. The final decision will depend on the anaesthetist's clinical judgement.
© Obstetric Anaesthetists' Association / Difficult Airway Society 2015)

Figure 8a.3 Decision-making tool for proceeding with surgery (reproduced with permission from Obstetric Anaesthetists' Association/Difficult Airway Society)

By practising this particular drill with the whole team, all members of the team will know where the difficult intubation trolley is kept. They will also gain a greater understanding of the reasons for requesting that the operation does not begin/continue and that theatre remains quiet while the anaesthetist ensures that ventilation of the woman is restored using the most appropriate method possible.

It may also be an appropriate time to discuss the importance of the close monitoring and surveillance that is required during extubation, and also for recovery of the woman after a general anaesthetic. Women can still be at risk from airway and respiratory complications during their recovery from general anaesthesia. The maternal mortality reports in the UK include women who have died from respiratory failure after general anaesthetic for caesarean section. Therefore, pregnant or postpartum women who undergo general anaesthesia require the same standards of staffing and monitoring as for recovery procedures in the non-pregnant population. It is important that the maternity staff caring for women who have undergone a general anaesthetic are trained in theatre recovery, and are able to maintain their competencies through regular sessions in general theatre recovery.

NOTE: There are further algorithms included on the Difficult Airway Society website, which may be recommended for use by your local anaesthetic department.[2] If this is the case, then it is important that these DAS algorithms are used in your training sessions.

Failed intubation scenario: clinical checklist

		Time	✓
Initial assessment (prior to general anaesthetic)	Good head position		
	Check cricoid position		
Preparation	Communicate with anaesthetic assistant, and pre-induction plan made with team (e.g. wake up or proceed in event of failed intubation)		
	Equipment and suction immediately to hand		
Pre-oxygenation	Appropriate technique and for appropriate length of time (aim $FiO_2 \geq 0.9$)		
Rapid sequence induction	Optimise position – head up/ramping		
	Consider facemask ventilation (P_{max} 20 cm H_2O)		
Laryngoscopy	After 1st attempt at intubation optimise view (e.g. reposition head, adjust cricoid pressure)		
	Maximum 2 attempts (3rd only by experienced colleague)		
Recognise the problem	Declare failed intubation to anaesthetic and obstetric team		
	Call for senior anaesthetist		
Maintain oxygenation	Release cricoid to insert supraglottic device		
	Supraglottic device (max 2 attempts to insert or facemask ± Guedel)		
Can't intubate, can't ventilate	Declare CICO to team		
	100% oxygen		
	Ensure adequate neuromuscular blockade		
Front of neck	Perform front of neck with scalpel, bougie and endotracheal tube		
Wake or proceed	Decision based on overall risk/benefit		
	Follow OAA-DAS algorithm accordingly		
Cardiac arrest	Institute BLS/ALS		
	Perimortem caesarean section		
Documentation	Timings, medication given, persons present		

Failed intubation scenario: teamwork checklists

Communication		YES	NO
State the problem	Clinical problem was stated clearly to arriving team		
Instructions	Instructions were clearly worded		
	Unnecessary conversation/noise was avoided		
	Action plans were shared		
Addressed	Specific instructions were given to the appropriate team members		
Sent	Communication was not rushed		
	It was clear what action was required		
Heard	Acknowledgements were made		
	Requests for repeat information were made		
Understood	The information was understood and repeated back by recipient		
	The correct action was performed		

Team roles and leadership		YES	NO
Roles	Each team member had a clear role		
	There was a team leader		
Adaptability	Team members responded well to different situations		
Responsibility	Team members assumed responsibility for their role		
Advocate	Tasks were delegated appropriately		
Feedback	There were regular updates on progress		
	A running commentary was provided		
Support	Team members did not argue about issues		
	None of the team members decided to 'go it alone'		

Section 8b: Cardiac arrest following local anaesthetic toxicity

> ## Key learning points
>
> Please refer to the learning points listed in **Section 7** (*Maternal cardiac arrest and advanced life support*), as these are also relevant to this scenario.
>
> The specific learning points for local anaesthetic (LA) toxicity are:
>
> - Management of severe local anaesthetic toxicity using AAGBI guideline.
> - Recognising that arrhythmias secondary to LA toxicity may be refractory to treatment, and that recovery from LA-induced cardiac arrest may take more than 1 hour.

Common difficulties observed in training drills

Again, please refer to the common difficulties listed in Section 7, as these are also relevant to this scenario.

The specific common difficulties for this scenario are:

- Not moving the bed away from the wall or removing the headboard
- Lack of knowledge of the use (or location) of Intralipid in the management of LA toxicity
- Focusing on specific management of LA toxicity and forgetting to exclude other causes of maternal cardiac arrest (e.g. hypovolaemia)
- Forgetting that perimortem birth can be achieved vaginally with forceps (and does not have to be by caesarean section) if the woman is fully dilated
- Not planning for a prolonged resuscitation

Aims of the local anaesthetic toxicity scenario

During this scenario the team should recognise cardiac arrest, call for appropriate help (including the maternal cardiac arrest team), immediately commence basic life support and move on to advanced life support as soon as possible. Staff should defibrillate the woman as soon as they are able, recognise that LA toxicity is a possible cause of the cardiac arrest and treat with intravenous Intralipid. As the woman is fully dilated and the presenting part is low, obstetric forceps can be used to assist the birth of the baby within 5 minutes.

Supporting material

The downloadable supporting materials included are:

- Treatment algorithms for basic and advanced life support
- Treatment algorithms and instructions for the treatment of LA toxicity
- Partogram and maternity notes
- Examples of ECG strips: sinus rhythm, ventricular tachycardia, ventricular fibrillation, asystole
- Pictures of automated external defibrillator (AED)
- Picture of a bag of Intralipid
- Pathological CTG

These are all in a printable format for use in the scenario.

Local anaesthetic toxicity (advanced life support) scenario

In this scenario, a labouring woman is given an epidural top-up so that she will be comfortable for an operative vaginal birth in the room (for a pathological CTG in the second stage). Immediately following the epidural top-up, the woman becomes agitated and then collapses. The scenario enables staff and students to practise basic and advanced life support (including defibrillation) in a pregnant woman who is fully dilated, and also enables the recognition and management of local anaesthetic toxicity to be practised and discussed.

An additional scenario that covers advanced life support is presented in
Section 7, relating to a woman who is undergoing induction of labour and
has a cardiac arrest secondary to a suspected amniotic fluid embolism (there
is a non-shockable rhythm in this scenario).

'This is Susan [a patient-mannequin] and her partner Roger [the second
drill facilitator]. This is her first pregnancy, and she has been induced
today following an uncomplicated pregnancy as she is 40^{+12} weeks. She
is normally fit and well, doesn't take any regular medication and has no
allergies. IV Syntocinon was commenced at 10.15 am this morning, and
Susan had an epidural sited at 11.30 am. It had been working well until
about 30 minutes ago.

Susan is in the second stage of labour and has been pushing for 15
minutes, but as you can see the CTG is pathological. The obstetrician
has just assessed her and is happy to perform an operative vaginal
birth (OVB) in the room. He has just gone to get the OVB trolley. The
anaesthetist has suggested I give 10 mL of 0.5% L-bupivacaine to top
up the epidural. I have literally just given it now. Are you OK to do a set
of observations for me, while I go and find out how long the doctor will
be? Thanks.'

The handover is given to a midwife in the room. Susan (the mannequin) is in
the lithotomy position and is pushing with contractions. Immediately after
the handover, the birth partner says that Susan is feeling really unwell and is
becoming agitated. Within a minute she has arrested.

The cardiac arrest should be managed as outlined in the advanced life
support scenario (Section 7). However, in this scenario (because the cardiac
arrest is caused by LA toxicity), when the defibrillator is attached there is
a shockable rhythm (ventricular fibrillation) and therefore defibrillation is
required.

As in any maternal cardiac arrest, the team should make immediate plans to
assist the birth of the baby, and this should be achieved within 5 minutes. In
this scenario, because the woman is fully dilated and the presenting part is
low, an operative vaginal birth (OVB) should be performed.

Ideally, Susan should recover only after she has been defibrillated
twice, the baby has been born and Intralipid has been administered

intravenously. However, some maternity staff may be unfamiliar with the use of Intralipid in the management of LA toxicity, and the drill facilitator may therefore 'allow' Susan to recover following defibrillation combined with the birth of the baby. The use of Intralipid can then be discussed in the debrief.

Equipment

- Full-body mannequin, e.g. SimMom (Laerdal, Norway) or Noelle (Gaumard), or a basic resuscitation mannequin such as Resusci-Anne
  - ☐ Fetus placed into the pelvis so that it is cephalic, below the spines and in a direct occipito-anterior (OA) position if using full-body mannequin
  - ☐ Wig, bra, pants, cushion and baby doll if using Resusci-Anne, or you could use PROMPT Flex birthing simulator as the bottom half of the mannequin for OVB
- IV access in situ, with IV fluids and pretend Syntocinon infusion connected to woman
- Empty 10 mL syringe labelled 0.5% L-bupivacaine (or the local anaesthetic used for top-up in your unit) and an empty 'ampoule' to check
- Cardiac arrest trolley (training trolley and drugs if possible):
  - ☐ Guedel airway
  - ☐ bag and mask
  - ☐ intubation equipment
  - ☐ medications (1 mg adrenaline – use 10 mL syringes labelled 'adrenaline')
  - ☐ IV cannulae with needles removed
  - ☐ IV crystalloid and giving sets
  - ☐ blood bottles and forms
  - ☐ stethoscope
- Perimortem caesarean section kit (or photograph)
- Defibrillator and pads
  - ☐ training AED (if available), programmed not to shock
  - ☐ or a cardboard-box defibrillator (see Appendix 3)

- Laminated 'bag' of Intralipid stored in its usual location (e.g. on the arrest trolley)
- Laminated ECG cardiac arrest rhythms: ventricular fibrillation, ventricular tachycardia, sinus rhythm, asystole
- CTG machine with laminated paper showing a pathological CTG
- Operative vaginal birth trolley containing non-rotational forceps
- Pillow and sheet
- Partogram, epidural chart and drug chart
- Laminated advanced life support algorithm
- Laminated algorithm for management of severe local anaesthetic toxicity
- Laminated clinical and teamwork checklists, with pens

Setting-up instructions

The drill should involve your hospital's resuscitation training department and/ or an obstetric anaesthetist for the training of advanced life support.

- Make sure the mannequin is dressed and has a pregnant abdomen containing a baby positioned in a cephalic presentation, below the spines and in a direct OA position.
- Place the mannequin into lithotomy position (ready for an OVB) and cover her with a sheet.
- 'Cannulate' the mannequin with a needleless IV cannula and attach a bag of crystalloid and a pretend Syntocinon infusion.
- Attach a CTG machine with the pathological CTG.
- Have a blood pressure cuff and stethoscope available.
- Prepare an OVB trolley, making sure there is a pair of non-rotational forceps available.
- The birth partner can push the baby through the mannequin for the OVB.
- Prepare a training cardiac arrest trolley containing the equipment outlined above. Clearly label this 'TRAINING CARDIAC ARREST TROLLEY' and if possible place this near the real cardiac arrest trolley, so that participants have to know where the actual trolley is kept. If you are training away from the clinical area, have the trolley nearby outside the room.

- If you are using a training AED, make sure you have programmed it to recognise a shockable rhythm and require at least two shocks when it is attached to the mannequin.

- Ensure that the partogram and maternity notes have been printed off, and use local epidural, medication and fluid charts.

Instructions for drill facilitators

The drill facilitator should give the handover to one member of the team. If there is a team observing the drill, they should stand in the corner of the room to observe the scenario; two of the team can be allocated to mark the clinical and teamwork checklists.

Following the handover, the facilitator should also stand in the corner of the room. If there is no other team observing, either the trainer or another of the drill facilitators completes the clinical and teamworking (communication and roles and responsibilities) checklists. The birth partner will then start saying that Susan is not behaving like her usual self.

If the observations are taken within the first minute tell the participants they are:

- Heart rate: 102 bpm
- Blood pressure 92/75 mmHg

As specific team members are requested to help, the trainer should go to the door and ask them to attend the emergency. If the emergency buzzer is used, all the team members should be asked to attend.

Participants should manually displace the mannequin's uterus to the left and refer to the basic and advanced life support algorithms in the *Course Manual* (Figure 8b.1).

If you are not using a pre-programmed training AED but your unit uses an AED, say, 'shock advised'. If your unit uses a manual defibrillator, show the laminated example of ventricular fibrillation (Figure 8b.2). Two shocks will be required before there is a return of circulation. After two shocks have been given and the baby has been born, the drill facilitator should explain that Susan has started to cough and move. Show the laminated example of sinus rhythm (Figure 8b.3), and this will conclude the scenario.

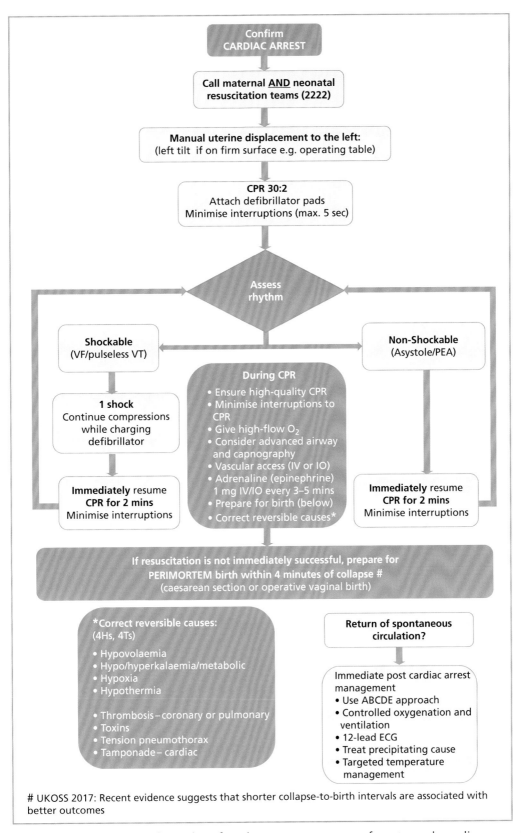

Figure 8b.1 Adapted algorithm for the management of maternal cardiac arrest (based on Resuscitation Council (UK) Guidelines, 2015)

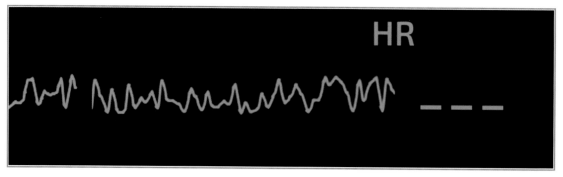

Figure 8b.2 Example of ventricular fibrillation

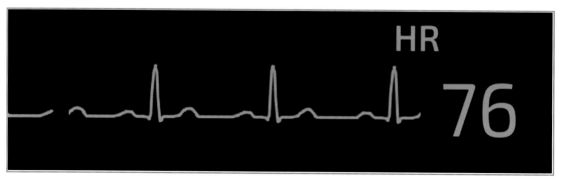

Figure 8b.3 Example of sinus rhythm

Prompts

Below are some suggestions to prompt the team if they are struggling with the scenario:

If collapse not noted:	'Is she OK?'
If help not called:	'Do you need some help?'
If CPR not commenced:	'Is there anything you should be starting?'
If the defibrillator is not attached:	'What is her heart rhythm doing?'
If an instrumental birth is not considered:	'What about the baby?'
If the neonatal team are not called:	'Who is going to look after the baby?'
If Intralipid is not commenced:	'Do you think the epidural top-up had anything to do with the cardiac arrest?'

Debrief and feedback

The debrief should cover all points regarding maternal cardiac arrest as outlined in Section 7.

Remember to discuss how staff can make the resuscitation easier by moving the bed into the centre of the room, removing the head of the bed and using the 'CPR handle' to immediately flatten the bed.

The recognition and management of local anaesthetic toxicity should be discussed. Talk together about the signs and symptoms of local anaesthetic toxicity, as outlined in the box.

Signs and symptoms of local anaesthetic toxicity

Warning signs	<ul><li>Tingling (lips/mouth/tongue)</li><li>Metallic taste in the mouth</li><li>Ringing in the ears</li><li>Light-headedness</li><li>Agitation ('just not right')</li><li>Tremor</li></ul>	
Severe toxicity	Neurological	Cardiovascular
	<ul><li>Severe agitation</li><li>Convulsions</li><li>Loss of consciousness</li></ul>	<ul><li>Bradycardia</li><li>Heart block</li><li>Asystole/cardiac arrest</li><li>Ventricular tachyarrhythmias</li></ul>

In the situation of suspected local anaesthetic toxicity, CPR should be combined with treatment with intravenous Intralipid. Explain to participants that they would not be expected to remember the dose of Intralipid required, as there will be instructions attached to the bag (Figure 8b.4), but they will need to know where it is kept and that it should be used in a cardiac arrest following suspected local anaesthetic toxicity.

During the debrief it should also be stressed that resuscitation from LA-induced cardiac arrest may take more than 1 hour, even when lipid emulsion is used. For this reason, the airway should be secured with an endotracheal tube to allow continuous chest compressions. The latter is very tiring; the team leader should continually assess the quality of chest compressions and ensure the team rotates this role frequently.

It should be stressed that whatever the cause of the cardiac arrest, the initial management is the same: early recognition, immediate chest compressions, followed by ventilation, defibrillation as soon as possible (if indicated), IV access and IV adrenaline. Once good-quality advanced life support is under way, the cause of the arrest should be considered (e.g. What was happening

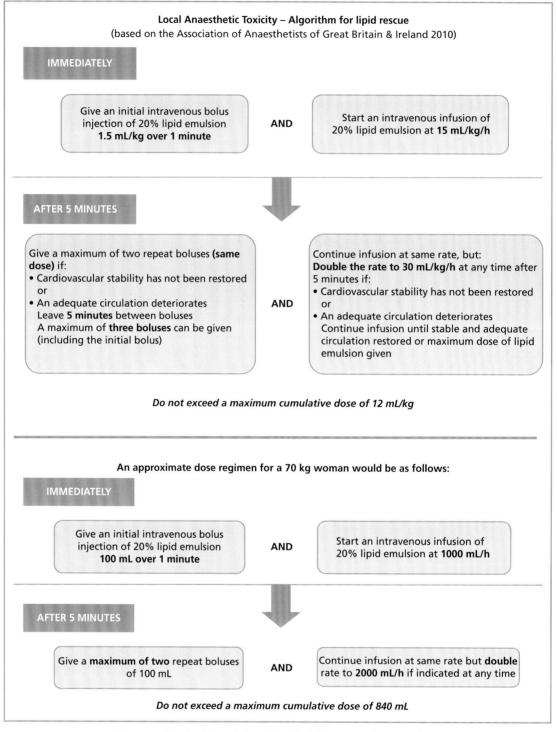

Local Anaesthetic Toxicity – Algorithm for lipid rescue
(based on the Association of Anaesthetists of Great Britain & Ireland 2010)

IMMEDIATELY

Give an initial intravenous bolus injection of 20% lipid emulsion **1.5 mL/kg over 1 minute**

AND

Start an intravenous infusion of 20% lipid emulsion at **15 mL/kg/h**

AFTER 5 MINUTES

Give a maximum of two repeat boluses **(same dose)** if:
• Cardiovascular stability has not been restored or
• An adequate circulation deteriorates
Leave **5 minutes** between boluses
A maximum of **three boluses** can be given (including the initial bolus)

AND

Continue infusion at same rate, but:
Double the rate to 30 mL/kg/h at any time after 5 minutes if:
• Cardiovascular stability has not been restored or
• An adequate circulation deteriorates
Continue infusion until stable and adequate circulation restored or maximum dose of lipid emulsion given

Do not exceed a maximum cumulative dose of 12 mL/kg

An approximate dose regimen for a 70 kg woman would be as follows:

IMMEDIATELY

Give an initial intravenous bolus injection of 20% lipid emulsion **100 mL over 1 minute**

AND

Start an intravenous infusion of 20% lipid emulsion at **1000 mL/h**

AFTER 5 MINUTES

Give a **maximum of two** repeat boluses of 100 mL

AND

Continue infusion at same rate but **double** rate to **2000 mL/h** if indicated at any time

Do not exceed a maximum cumulative dose of 840 mL

Figure 8b.4 Algorithm for lipid rescue (AAGBI)

immediately prior to the arrest? What is the woman's past medical history? Is the woman bleeding?). Specific treatment can then be given, in conjunction with CPR, to address the cause of the collapse (e.g. Intralipid for LA toxicity as described above, IV fluid and blood in the case of haemorrhage, 10 mL of 10% calcium gluconate in the case of magnesium toxicity).

Local anaesthetic toxicity scenario: clinical checklist

		Time	✓
Recognise problem	Call for help		
	Emergency buzzer activated		
	Call 2222 and state 'maternal cardiac arrest' (include neonatal team)		
Equipment	Ask for cardiac arrest trolley		
Position of mother	Keep mother supine and manually displace uterus to the left		
Assess	Check own safety to approach		
	Check responsiveness		
Airway	Open airway		
	Secure airway		
Breathing	Assess breathing and observe for signs of life for up to 10 seconds (look, listen, feel)		
	If not breathing, start chest compressions		
Circulation	Chest compressions at ratio 30:2, rate 100–120 per minute		
	Attach defibrillator/monitor and assess rhythm		
IV access	Insert 2nd IV cannula and take bloods		
Reversible causes verbalised	4 H's and 4 T's (see *Course Manual*, Module 3)		
	Toxins – local anaesthetic toxicity		
Specific management	Lipid emulsion bolus given		
	Lipid emulsion infusion commenced		
Documentation	Timings		
	Medication given		
	Persons present		

Local anaesthetic toxicity scenario: teamwork checklists

Communication		YES	NO
State the problem	Clinical problem was stated clearly to arriving team		
Instructions	Instructions were clearly worded		
	Unnecessary conversation/noise was avoided		
	Action plans were shared		
	Goals were clearly identified		
Addressed	Specific instructions were given to the appropriate team members		
Sent	Communication was not rushed		
	It was clear what action was required		
Heard	Acknowledgements were made		
	Requests for repeat information were made		
Understood	The information was understood and repeated back by recipient		
	The correct action was performed		

Team roles and leadership		YES	NO
Roles	Each team member had a clear role		
	There was a team leader		
Adaptability	Team members responded well to different situations		
Responsibility	Team members assumed responsibility for their role		
Advocate	Tasks were delegated appropriately		
Feedback	There were regular updates on progress		
	A running commentary was provided		
Support	Team members did not argue about issues		
	None of the team members decided to 'go it alone'		

Section 8c: Total spinal block

Key learning points

■ ABC approach to resuscitation.

■ To understand the possible serious adverse effects of epidurals.

Common difficulties observed in training drills

■ Forgetting either to put the mother into full left-lateral position or to use left uterine displacement or left tilt

■ Not being aware of the possibility and effects of total spinal block

Aims of the total spinal block scenario

The main aim of this scenario is to emphasise that, whatever the cause of maternal collapse, resuscitation should follow the basic ABC (airway, breathing, circulation) protocol. The secondary aim is to remind all maternity staff of one of the potential serious adverse effects of epidural anaesthesia.

Supporting material

The downloadable supporting materials included are:

■ Treatment algorithm for total spinal block

■ Maternity notes

■ Partogram

■ ECGs: sinus bradycardia and sinus rhythm

■ CTG and CTG pro forma

These are all in a printable format for use in the scenario.

Total spinal block scenario

This scenario presents a woman in her first pregnancy requiring an operative vaginal birth (OVB) for a pathological cardiotocograph (CTG). The obstetrician decides that the procedure can be carried out in the labour ward room and therefore the anaesthetist administers a strong epidural top-up for pain relief. A total spinal block occurs and the team is required to support and assist the anaesthetist in managing this rare but very acute emergency. The scenario enables anaesthetists, theatre staff, obstetricians, midwives and healthcare support workers to gain experience of the immediate management of a total spinal block, and also the teamworking required when this situation occurs. Management should include recognising the problem and relaying this to the whole team, calling for help and following the total spinal block algorithm.

'This is Mary [a patient-mannequin]. She is 32 years old, has no past medical history, and this is her first pregnancy. She has had no problems in her pregnancy but has had to undergo induction of labour for being post-term at 40 weeks + 12 days.

She is on the labour ward and had an epidural sited 2 hours after starting a Syntocinon infusion to induce labour. She has progressed well and is now fully dilated. She has been pushing for 2 hours but is now getting tired and there is a pathological CTG. The vertex is just visible, but Mary feels she can't push any longer. The obstetrician is concerned about the fetal condition and has therefore recommended that Mary be given assistance to give birth. Mary has agreed to an operative vaginal birth (OVB) and the obstetrician is confident that the procedure can be safely carried out in the labour ward room.

Mary is starting to feel pain and the obstetrician asks the anaesthetist if he could administer adequate pain relief so that she is comfortable during an OVB in the room.

The anaesthetist informs the anaesthetic assistant that they are doing the procedure in the room and then gives Mary an epidural top-up of 10 mL of 0.5% L-bupivacaine. You are now preparing for the OVB.'

Equipment

- Full-body mannequin, e.g. SimMom (Laerdal, Norway), or a basic resuscitation mannequin such as Resusci-Anne:
  - ☐ fetus placed into the pelvis so that it is cephalic, below the spines and direct OA if using full-body mannequin
  - ☐ wig, bra, pants, cushion and baby doll if using Resusci-Anne, or you could use a PROMPT Flex birthing simulator for the bottom half of the mannequin for the operative vaginal birth
- Needleless intravenous cannula taped to arm with infusion (1 L crystalloid) attached and also Syntocinon infusion
- Syringe labelled 'Syntocinon infusion' connected to patient
- Pillows – maximum two
- CTG belts and transducers
- CTG machine (a real one, or a cardboard box with pictures on)
- CTG traces showing (a) prolonged fetal bradycardia and (b) pathological CTG
- Epidural catheter and filter
- Blood pressure cuff and machine (or laminated picture)
- Simple (Hudson) oxygen mask and oxygen mask with reservoir bag
- Bag-valve-mask system (e.g. Ambu bag) for ventilation
- Laryngoscope, endotracheal tubes (7.0, 7.5 and 8.0), tube tie, 10 mL syringe to inflate balloon
- Laryngeal mask (size 4)
- Needleless intravenous cannulae of various sizes
- Intravenous fluids of various types including crystalloid as used in your unit (two bags of each)
- 1–2 × 20 mL syringe labelled 'thiopental' or 'propofol' as used in your unit
- 2 × 2 mL syringe labelled 'suxamethonium', or 5–10 mL syringe labelled 'rocuronium'
- Syringes labelled for vasopressors (e.g. ephedrine, phenylephrine, metaraminol) as used in your unit
- 10 mL syringe labelled '0.5% L-bupivacaine' (or the local anaesthetic mix used for top-ups in your unit) and empty ampoule to check (could be a re-labelled normal saline vial)
- Defibrillator and pads

- Laminated ECG showing sinus bradycardia and one showing normal heart rate
- Stethoscope
- Operative vaginal birth trolley containing non-rotational forceps and cord clamps as a minimum
- Partogram, maternity notes and locally used epidural chart
- Laminated clinical and teamwork checklists, with pens

Setting-up instructions

Ideally, the scenario would be run in an actual labour ward room, so that staff are familiar with the equipment. If you do not want the team to know what the scenario is going to be, you may wish to call this a 'category 1 operative vaginal birth' drill.

- The woman (mannequin) should be lying semi-recumbent on a bed wearing a hospital gown or T-shirt. She should have one IV cannula in place on her arm with IV fluids attached and Syntocinon infusion. The mannequin should have an epidural catheter and filter secured with tape over her shoulder.
- A CTG machine (cardboard-box CTG machine) is attached with a pathological trace showing a baseline of 150 bpm and atypical variable decelerations. Further sections of CTG should be available showing a prolonged fetal bradycardia, which can be used when the woman loses consciousness.
- Ensure that general anaesthetic drugs and vasopressors are available in the usual place (e.g. fridge).
- Ensure that intubation equipment is available.
- Ensure maternity notes, partogram and locally used epidural chart are available.
- Have an empty ampoule of 10 mL 0.5% L-bupivacaine (simulate this with a 10 mL normal saline vial) and a syringe labelled '0.5% L-bupivacaine' containing 10 mL of saline or water.
- Construct a training resuscitation trolley or use the one in your department (ensuring that everyone in the department is aware that you are using it and that the location is clearly identified).
- Instruments should be available for performing an OVB, although the emphasis for this scenario is on the treatment of the high spinal block.

Instructions for drill facilitators

This drill should be led by an experienced anaesthetist.

A handover about Mary (the patient-mannequin) should be given to a midwife, an anaesthetist and an obstetrician as outlined above. Other anaesthetic staff could also be included.

The obstetrician, midwife, neonatologist and healthcare assistant/midwifery assistant participants should assume their usual roles during the preparation for an OVB.

If a team is observing the drill, they should stand in the corner of the labour ward room to observe the scenario; two of the team can be allocated to mark the clinical and teamwork checklists.

The scenario begins with the anaesthetist giving an epidural top-up of 10 mL of 0.5% L-bupivacaine. Very quickly, Mary complains of feeling dizzy and a bit sick. One of the faculty may act as Mary's 'voiceover' or as her birthing partner. After approximately 1 minute she says she is having difficulty breathing and feels terrible. Soon after, she loses consciousness and stops breathing. She still has a pulse, which feels weak, and a measurable blood pressure.

Over the course of the scenario, Mary will become unconscious, have an increasingly low blood pressure, have an initially fast pulse that will then become very slow, have low oxygen saturations, and will eventually stop breathing.

The anaesthetist is expected to recognise the problem and organise the team to take an ABC approach to resuscitating Mary. Help should be called immediately. The woman should be laid flat with left uterine displacement or left tilt using a wedge. The team should administer high-flow oxygen, ventilate the woman and then intubate the trachea, give fast IV fluids and support blood pressure with vasopressors. The legs should be elevated if possible.

The obstetrician should await instructions from the anaesthetist as to when they can continue with the instrumental birth. The scenario ends when the baby is born and all the above resuscitative measures have been undertaken. The woman will not arrest unless no resuscitative measures are undertaken.

Encourage the participants to call for help early on and follow the management of total spinal block algorithm (use your local guideline or the example in Figure 8c.1).

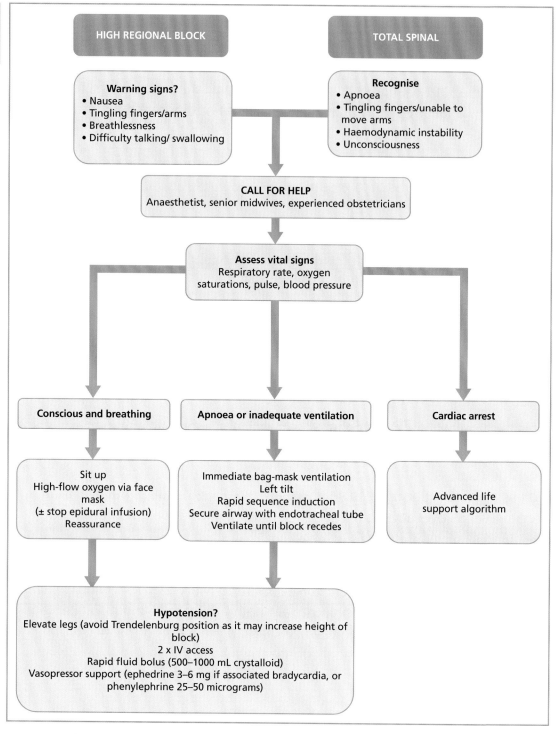

Figure 8c.1 Algorithm for the management of total spinal block

Once immediate resuscitation has taken place and the patient has a secure airway and is being ventilated, she will need to be transferred to theatre/ ICU. She will require continued ventilatory and circulatory support with appropriate sedation until the total spinal block wears off and adequate spontaneous breathing resumes.

> **It is important that the team is supported by the facilitators sufficiently so that Mary survives, making it a positive experience for the participants.**

Prompts

Listed below are the observations and responses if team members ask for information:

Initial observations			
Pulse:	95 bpm	Mary:	'I feel a bit dizzy and a bit sick.'
Blood pressure:	90/50 mmHg	CTG:	pathological
1 minute later			
Pulse:	110 bpm	Mary:	'I feel really terrible and I can't breathe.'
Blood pressure:	80/40 mmHg	CTG:	bradycardia
At 2 minutes			
Pulse:	45 bpm	Mary:	unresponsive and not breathing
Blood pressure:	70/35 mmHg	CTG:	bradycardia
Oxygen saturation (SpO$_2$):	Falling		

The observations will gradually improve as fluid, vasopressors, oxygen and ventilatory support are given.

Participant question	Drill facilitator response	
'Is she breathing?'	Before loss of consciousness:	YES
	After loss of consciousness:	NO
'Are there any signs of an allergic reaction?'	No obvious redness or wheezing	
'Is there any bleeding?'	No blood can be seen (*make sure the participants have actually looked*)	
'Is the baby alright?'	*Show the CTG trace of persistent bradycardia*	

Debrief and feedback

Ideally, the scenario is run with the multi-professional team so that communication between all members of the team is encouraged. Use the clinical and communication checklists to aid the debrief.

Emphasise the importance of following the basic ABC (airway, breathing, circulation) protocol, irrespective of the cause of maternal collapse.

Include discussions on epidural anaesthesia and its potential serious adverse effects. This may also lead on to discussions about the decision to perform the operative vaginal birth in the labour ward room and not transferring the woman to theatre.

By practising this particular drill with the whole team, all team members will gain a greater understanding of the reasons for requesting that preparations for the operative vaginal birth cease (irrespective of the fetal condition), and that staff should remain quiet while the anaesthetist ensures that the woman's condition is stabilised and ventilation is restored using the most appropriate method possible.

References

1. Obstetric Anaesthetists' Association, Difficult Airway Society. OAA DAS obstetric airway guidelines 2015. www.oaa-anaes.ac.uk/ui/content/content.aspx?id=3447 (accessed August 2017).
2. Difficult Airway Society. Guidelines for the management of difficult and failed tracheal intubation in obstetrics – 2015. https://www.das.uk.com/guidelines/obstetric_airway_guide-lines_2015 (accessed August 2017).

Total spinal block scenario: clinical checklist

		Time	✓
Recognise problem`	Call for help		
	Emergency buzzer activated		
Assess	Check own safety to approach		
	Check responsiveness		
Airway	Is woman talking?		
	If not, open airway		
Breathing	Assess breathing		
	Give oxygen at 15 litres/minute via mask with reservoir bag		
	Ventilate with bag-valve-mask and/or secure airway when stops breathing		
Circulation	Check pulse and blood pressure		
	Give IV fluids		
	Left uterine displacement or left tilt		
	Give vasopressors and elevate legs		
IV access	Insert second IV cannula and take bloods		
Documentation	Timings		
	Medication given		
	Persons present		

Total spinal block scenario: teamwork checklists

Communication		YES	NO
State the problem	Clinical problem was stated clearly to arriving team		
Instructions	Instructions were clearly worded		
	Unnecessary conversation/noise was avoided		
	Action plans were shared		
	Goals were clearly identified		
Addressed	Specific instructions were given to the appropriate team members		
Sent	Communication was not rushed		
	It was clear what action was required		
Heard	Acknowledgements were made		
	Requests for repeat information were made		
Understood	The information was understood and repeated back by recipient		
	The correct action was performed		

Team roles and leadership		YES	NO
Roles	Each team member had a clear role		
	There was a team leader		
Adaptability	Team members responded well to different situations		
Responsibility	Team members assumed responsibility for their role		
Advocate	Tasks were delegated appropriately		
Feedback	There were regular updates on progress		
	A running commentary was provided		
Support	Team members did not argue about issues		
	None of the team members decided to 'go it alone'		

Section 9
Fetal monitoring in labour

Key learning points

- On admission in labour, a full clinical and obstetric risk assessment should be undertaken to determine the most appropriate method of fetal monitoring. Risk assessments should continue throughout labour to identify any indications for transferring to continuous electronic fetal monitoring (EFM).

- Healthy women with an uncomplicated pregnancy should be offered and recommended intermittent auscultation in labour.

- Continuous EFM should be offered and recommended for women with antenatal and/or intrapartum risk factors.

- A CTG should always be interpreted holistically, in context with the medical, clinical and obstetric circumstances as well as the woman's preferences, when determining the appropriate actions to be taken.

- Excessive uterine activity is the most frequent cause of fetal hypoxia/acidosis.

- It is best practice for all maternity staff to record their opinion and actions clearly and legibly using a structured pro forma at least hourly, and to obtain a timely 'fresh eyes' review.

Problems identified from case discussions

- Not auscultating the fetal heart rate for a full minute, starting towards the end of the contraction and continuing for at least 30 seconds after the contraction has ended (FIGO) *OR* not auscultating the fetal heart rate immediately after a contraction (NICE)

- Not documenting a systematic assessment of the CTG at least hourly, and at each review

- Interpreting the CTG in isolation and not considering the full clinical picture

- Not seeking help from experienced practitioners from the multi-professional team to assist with decision making when the CTG is difficult to interpret

- Not continuing/recommencing EFM when transferring a mother to theatre to expedite the birth

Introduction to CTG interpretation and multi-professional training

Poor recognition of CTG abnormalities, and failure to take appropriate action once abnormalities have been detected, have been identified almost ubiquitously by national reports for nearly two decades, without any clear improvements.[1,2,3,4] Clearly, these important failings in 'human' factors have contributed to the poor outcomes.

The recent *Saving Babies' Lives* care bundle, published in 2016 by NHS England,[5] includes a chapter on 'Effective fetal monitoring in labour' as one of the four key elements outlined in the document. Their rationale for including this element is that '*CTG interpretation requires a high level of skill and is susceptible to variation in judgment between clinicians ... and can lead to inappropriate care ... subsequently impacting on perinatal outcomes.*' The care bundle also recommends that NHS Trusts must demonstrate that all qualified staff who care for women in labour are competent to interpret CTGs, and they must identify appropriate training packages to ensure clinical competence. However, there is no clear guidance as to how this should be achieved.

In 2011, a systematic review of CTG training concluded that training can improve CTG competence and clinical practice, but that further research is needed to evaluate the type and content of training that is most effective.[6] This has been borne out by two recent national patient safety programmes in Sweden and Denmark, which included screen-based CTG training but were not associated with any improvements in perinatal outcomes.[7,8,9]

Mandatory multi-professional skills training in CTG interpretation and obstetric emergencies has been associated with improvements in neonatal outcomes in the UK[10] and replicated in Kansas, USA,[11] and Victoria, Australia.[12] Training covered CTG interpretation and also the skills required to communicate the interpretation and the actions of the team responding to the emergency. We consider it likely that improving outcomes in labour when EFM is used requires more than just isolated CTG interpretation training, and that it should include appropriate technical and non-technical skills, including team skills.[4]

Running the session

Given the communication skills requirement for facilitating CTG interpretation, and the interactive nature of the team response to any actions taken, it is a good idea for the fetal monitoring session to be conducted in an interactive group discussion format.

Trainers should read the PROMPT *Course Manual* chapter on fetal monitoring in labour (Module 5) prior to running their session, so that they are familiar with the most up-to-date national guidance and also the documentation aids that are used in both the CTG presentations and the case histories.

There are two CTG interpretation workbooks included in the downloadable supporting materials. The workbooks contain the first part of each of the case histories that are included in the PowerPoint presentations. The appropriate workbook can be distributed to the teams at the start of the fetal monitoring session, and they should be given approximately 15 minutes to review the case, document their opinions, actions and comments as a team.

Each case history has been selected to illustrate key learning points. We suggest it would be good to highlight that the information included in these case studies is based solely on standard documentation written in the maternity notes and partogram. If any information is missing, this could be used to emphasise the importance of making accurate and thorough documentation.

It is important to stress that classifying CTGs can be difficult, but that using the appropriate CTG pro formas can help both to standardise and to facilitate the classification across the entire multi-professional team,[13] and should be encouraged by all maternity staff in the unit. In addition, one of the most important factors of CTG interpretation is deciding what action should be taken based on the CTG classification, in the context of the clinical circumstances and the woman's preferences. Using the CTG pro formas will also facilitate this process and provide a written record for all staff to review.[13]

Downloadable PowerPoint presentations

In addition to the two case history presentations, there are five other PowerPoint presentations covering the different aspects of fetal monitoring guidance, interpretation and fetal physiology that can be downloaded and used in your fetal monitoring sessions. They are:

1. Fetal monitoring in labour – national guidelines and recommendations
2. Fetal monitoring in labour – fetal physiology
3. Fetal monitoring in labour – intermittent auscultation
4. Fetal monitoring in labour – electronic fetal monitoring
5. Interpreting antenatal CTGs

The choice of which presentations to use will depend on the length of time allocated to your *Fetal monitoring in labour* session, and also on which aspects are important to be taught locally. It may be that you wish to run a separate multi-professional workshop on fetal monitoring in labour (i.e. not as part of your local PROMPT course training day), in which case all presentations could be used and both of the case histories also incorporated into the workshop. However, if fetal monitoring in labour is included as one of the sessions on your local PROMPT day then there may only be enough time for a couple of the talks, e.g. fetal physiology plus EFM and intermittent auscultation, plus one of the case histories. In addition, you may wish to use the separate presentations for ad hoc short training sessions on the labour ward/birth centre, and also for student midwives and doctors.

All of the fetal monitoring in labour presentations are based on the FIGO 2015 fetal monitoring in labour guidelines,[14,15,16] and also the NICE 2014 intrapartum care guideline (including the updated fetal monitoring section released in March 2017).[17]

Downloadable documentation and CTG interpretation tools

There are examples of fetal monitoring pro formas that will be used throughout the sessions (Figures 9.1–9.6). They are based on information included in the FIGO consensus guidelines on fetal monitoring (2015)[14,15,16] and the revised NICE fetal monitoring guidance (2017).[17]

Intrapartum intermittent auscultation (IA)
Practice Recommendations (based on FIGO 2015)

Features to evaluate	Action	What to document
Fetal heart rate (FHR) (Normal: 110–160 bpm)	Duration: Listen for at least 60 seconds Timing: Listen towards the end of the contraction (as soon as it is comfortable for mother) and continue for at least 30 seconds after contraction Interval: 1st stage: every 15 minutes 2nd stage: every 5 minutes	• FHR as single number having counted for 60 seconds • Any slowing of FHR that may indicate decelerations or bradycardia • Any increase of FHR that may indicate fetal tachycardia
Uterine contractions	Palpate before and during FHR auscultation	• Number of contractions in 10 minutes
Fetal movements	Palpate at the same time as contractions The fetal heart rate may speed up in association with fetal movement	• Presence or absence of fetal movements • Any speeding up of FHR associated with fetal movement
Maternal pulse rate	At start of IA and at least hourly or if any FHR abnormality	• Maternal pulse as single counted number
If any abnormal features are identified, refer to: 'IA: Guidance and management if abnormal features identified in labour'		

Complete an intermittent auscultation (IA) pro forma on commencement of IA in labour and at handover of care during active labour

Record FHR and any required actions on the partogram

Figure 9.1 Practice recommendations for intermittent auscultation in labour

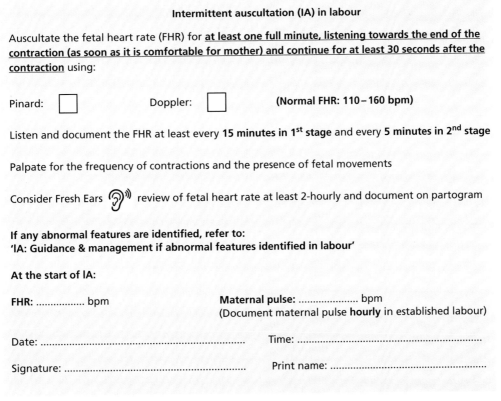

Intermittent auscultation (IA) in labour

Auscultate the fetal heart rate (FHR) for <u>**at least one full minute, listening towards the end of the contraction (as soon as it is comfortable for mother) and continue for at least 30 seconds after the contraction**</u> using:

Pinard: [ ]   Doppler: [ ]   **(Normal FHR: 110–160 bpm)**

Listen and document the FHR at least every **15 minutes in 1st stage** and every **5 minutes in 2nd stage**

Palpate for the frequency of contractions and the presence of fetal movements

Consider Fresh Ears 👂 review of fetal heart rate at least 2-hourly and document on partogram

If any abnormal features are identified, refer to:
'IA: Guidance & management if abnormal features identified in labour'

At the start of IA:

FHR: .... bpm   **Maternal pulse:** .... bpm
                                          (Document maternal pulse **hourly** in established labour)

Date: ....   Time: ....

Signature: ....   Print name: ....

Figure 9.2 An example of a pro forma used for documenting intermittent auscultation at the start of labour, with consideration for 2-hourly 'fresh ears' review

IA: Guidance and management if abnormal features identified in labour (based on FIGO 2015)

Features	Abnormal	Action
Fetal heart rate (FHR) (Normal: 110–160 bpm)	FHR less than 110 bpm	• Check maternal pulse rate and listen continuously to FHR. If FH remains at less than 110 bpm for more than 3 minutes, this suggests a prolonged deceleration or bradycardia • Change maternal position, perform VE, commence immediate CTG (if appropriate) and seek obstetric opinion • If at home, or in midwifery-led unit, arrange for immediate transfer to obstetric unit • In addition: if in the 2nd stage of labour and birth **not** immediately imminent, consider stopping pushing
	FHR less than 110 bpm for more than 5 minutes	• Expedite birth urgently
	FHR greater than 160 bpm	• Check maternal pulse rate and listen for 3 consecutive contractions - if still above 160 bpm suggestive of fetal tachycardia (NB. If fetal heart rate returns to normal range during this period, resume IA as per guidance for 1st or 2nd stage of labour) • Change maternal position, perform VE, commence continuous CTG, (if appropriate) and seek obstetric opinion • If at home, or in midwifery-led unit, arrange for immediate transfer to obstetric unit • Assess maternal temperature and for signs of infection
Fetal movements	An increasing FHR heard just after a contraction is rarely due to fetal movement	• IA should be carried out over the next 3 contractions to rule out the possibility of decelerations
Uterine contractions	An interval of less than 2 minutes between 2 contractions should trigger palpation over 10 minutes.	• If palpate more than 5 contractions in 10 minutes this indicates tachysystole • If tachysystole is indicated, commence continuous CTG (transfer to obstetric unit if necessary) and seek obstetric opinion • Consider tocolysis

Figure 9.3 Intermittent auscultation: guidance and management if abnormal features identified in labour

Antenatal CTG Pro forma	Reassuring	Non-reassuring	
Baseline rate (bpm)	110–160 Rate:	Less than 110 Rate: More than 160 Rate:	Comments:-
N.B Rising baseline rate even within normal range may be a concern if other non-reassuring features present			
Variability (bpm)	5 bpm or more	Less than 5 bpm for 50 minutes or more Sinusoidal pattern for 10 minutes or more Saltatory pattern of more than 25 bpm for 10 minutes or more	Comments:-
Accelerations	Present	None for 50 minutes	Comments:-
Decelerations	None	Unprovoked deceleration/s Decelerations related to uterine tightenings (not in labour)	Comments:-
Opinion	Normal CTG (All 4 features reassuring)	Abnormal CTG (1 or more non-reassuring features)	
Clinical information	Maternal pulse:	Membranes ruptured: Y/N If yes, date and time:	Liquor colour: Gestation (wks):

Reason for CTG:

Action: (An abnormal CTG requires prompt review by experienced obstetrician/senior midwife)

| Date: | Time: | Signature: .... Print: .... Designation: .... |

Figure 9.4 An example of an electronic fetal monitoring pro forma for use antenatally

Documentation pro forma for intrapartum CTG interpretation (based on FIGO 2015 and NICE 2017)			
Feature	**Reassuring (acceptable)**	**Non-reassuring**	**Abnormal**
Baseline rate (bpm)	Baseline 110 – 160 bpm Rate:	Baseline rate 100 – 109 bpm for **more than 10** minutes Baseline rate **more than 160 bpm for more than 10** minutes Rate:	Baseline **less than 100 bpm** Rate: Baseline rate **more than 180 bpm** Rate:
N.B A rising baseline rate even within the normal range may be of concern if other non-reassuring/abnormal features are present.			
Variability (bpm)	Variability of 5 – 25 bpm Comments:	Variability **less than 5 bpm for 30 to 50** minutes Variability **more than 25 bpm for 15 to 25** minutes	Variability **less than 5 bpm for more than 50** minutes Variability **more than 25 bpm for more than 25** minutes Sinusoidal pattern lasting for **more than 30** minutes
Accelerations	Present	Comments:	
Decelerations	None True early decelerations V-shaped variable decelerations (*NO concerning features*) with **less than 50%** of contractions NON V-shaped (U-shaped) variable decelerations (*NO concerning features*) with **more than 50%** of contractions for **less than 90** minutes NON V-shaped (U-shaped) variable decelerations with **less than 50%** of contractions *(and all other features of CTG are reassuring)*	V-shaped variable decelerations (*NO concerning features*) with **more than 50%** of contractions for **more than 90** minutes NON V-shaped (U-shaped) variable decelerations – (*concerning features present*) with **more than 50%** of contractions for **less than 30** minutes Repetitive **late** decelerations (U-shaped) for **less than 30** minutes Single prolonged deceleration lasting **more than 3** minutes, but **less than 5** minutes	NON V-shaped (U-shaped) variable decelerations – (*concerning features present*) with **more than 50%** of contractions and for **more than 30** minutes Repetitive **late** decelerations (U-shaped) for **more than 30** minutes Repetitive late decelerations (U-shaped) <u>and</u> reduced variability for **more than 20** minutes Single prolonged deceleration for **more than 5** minutes *(A prolonged deceleration of less than 80 bpm with reduced variability and lasting more than 5 minutes is often associated with hypoxia)*

Contractions :10 (N.B If more than 5:10 - take action to reduce frequency)	Dilatation:	Liquor colour:	Gestation:	Maternal pulse:
Reason for CTG:		Other risk factors:		

Opinion (N.B If CTG has any non-reassuring or abnormal features present from the start, it may not be appropriate to wait for specified time limits before requesting review)	**Normal CTG** (All *four* FHR features are reassuring) *No intervention necessary*	**Suspicious CTG** (*One* non-reassuring FHR feature) *Low probability of hypoxia* Correct reversible causes (refer to algorithm & EFM interpretation guidance)	**Pathological CTG** (*Two or more non-reassuring or one or more abnormal FHR features*) **High probability of hypoxia – urgent action required** (refer to algorithm & EFM Interpretation guidance)
Action taken: (Always consider the clinical circumstances when reviewing CTG and deciding action)			

Date: .... Time: .... Signature: .... Status: ....

at least 2 hourly

Time: .... Signature: .... Status: ....

Fresh Eyes Opinion   I agree with opinion? YES / NO   If opinion different complete new pro forma

Date: ....

NHS
North Bristol
NHS Trust

Figure 9.5 An example of an electronic fetal monitoring pro forma for use in labour

Intrapartum CTG classification, interpretation and action (based on FIGO 2015 and NICE 2017)	
Feature	**Information**
Baseline rate (bpm) The mean level of the FHR that is estimated over 10 minute periods	• May be necessary to review previous segments of CTG and/or evaluate the baseline over a longer period of time if there are episodes of unstable FHR patterns. Preterm fetuses have a faster heart rate • A bradycardia is a baseline rate below 110 bpm lasting for more than 10 minutes. Values between 100 and 110 bpm may be normal, especially in post term pregnancies, but in this instance, *all other features of the CTG will be reassuring* • Maternal pyrexia is the most common cause of fetal tachycardia (FHR more than 160 bpm)
Variability (bpm) The variability of the FHR signal as displayed via the CTG tracing	• Intermittent periods of reduced variability are normal, especially during periods of quiescence (sleep) • Reduced variability can occur due to central nervous system hypoxia • Increased variability (saltatory pattern) of greater than 25 bpm bandwidth for more than 25 minutes may indicate hypoxia
Sinusoidal pattern Smooth & undulating, resembling a sine wave with amplitude of 5 – 15 bpm. It lasts for more than 30 minutes and is absent of accelerations	• A sinusoidal pattern occurs in association with fetal anaemia and sometimes acute fetal hypoxia
Accelerations Abrupt increase in FHR of more than 15 bpm above the baseline, lasting longer than 15 seconds (but less than 10 minutes)	• Most accelerations coincide with fetal movement and are a sign that the fetus **is not hypoxic**. The absence of accelerations in an otherwise normal CTG is unlikely to indicate hypoxia/acidosis
Decelerations Decrease in the fetal heart rate of more than 15 bpm and lasting for more than 15 seconds	• **Early decelerations:** Short-lasting and shallow with normal variability within the decelerations, coinciding exactly with contractions – believed to be caused by head compression and does not indicate hypoxia • **Variable decelerations:** Varying in shape, size and relationship to contractions. Usually associated with cord compression V-shaped variable decelerations **(NO concerning features)** – exhibit a symmetrical rapid drop and rapid recovery to the baseline with good variability within deceleration *and all other features of the CTG are reassuring*. These seldom indicate hypoxia NON V-shaped/U-shaped variable decelerations (concerning features present i.e. **reduced variability within the deceleration)** *– these are highly likely to indicate hypoxia if they occur with more than 50% of contractions and continue for more than 30 minutes* • **Late decelerations:** Repetitive, U-shaped and/or with reduced variability within the deceleration and returning to baseline *after the end of the contraction*. Gradual onset and/or gradual return to baseline, starting more than 20 seconds after the onset of a contraction – *these are highly likely to indicate hypoxia* • **Prolonged deceleration:** Lasting more than 3 minutes but less than 5 minutes is non-reassuring. It is abnormal if it lasts more than 5 minutes. Expedite birth in shortest possible time if bradycardia persists beyond 5 minutes • **Decelerations of longer than 5 minutes with a FHR less than 80 bpm and reduced variability are often associated with hypoxia and urgent action is required**
Opinion & Actions: Always consider the medical, clinical & obstetric circumstances when interpreting the CTG and determining the actions to be taken If CTG has any non-reassuring or abnormal features present from the start, it may not be appropriate to wait for specified time limits before requesting review	**Normal:** No action required **Suspicious:** Correct reversible causes: Change position, inform midwife coordinator or obstetrician, reduce (or STOP) oxytocin infusion, perform VE if appropriate, assess maternal pulse, respiratory rate, B/P, temperature, check for signs of infection, continue to monitor FHR closely, consider additional methods to assess fetal oxygenation. **(Refer to Actions for Suspicious CTG Algorithm)** **Pathological:** Immediate actions to correct reversible causes, STOP oxytocin infusion, inform midwife coordinator and senior obstetrician, perform VE (if appropriate), exclude fetal hypoxia (Fetal Scalp Stimulation (FSS) and/or Fetal Blood Sampling (FBS) if possible & appropriate). If in the 2nd stage of labour and birth is not immediately imminent, consider stopping pushing. **If a severe or acute event is suspected, then an FBS is not advised as it may delay action. If fetal hypoxia confirmed or if further assessment of fetal oxygenation is not possible, take action to expedite birth. (Refer to Actions for Pathological CTG Algorithm)**

Figure 9.6 Summary of EFM guidance, interpretation and actions to be taken

All of the additional tools, documentation and cognitive aids included in the fetal monitoring training sessions can be printed from the downloadable materials and are listed below:

- Admission assessment for fetal monitoring in labour
- Intermittent auscultation practice recommendations
- Guidance if an abnormal fetal heart rate is suspected and identified in labour
- An example of an intermittent auscultation documentation pro forma (based on FIGO 2015)
- Example of an intrapartum CTG documentation pro forma
- Summary of guidance for intrapartum CTG classification, interpretation and action
- Suggested actions if CTG suspicious
- Suggested actions if CTG pathological

References

1. Cantwell R, Clutton-Brock T, Cooper G, *et al.* Saving Mothers' Lives: reviewing maternal deaths to make motherhood safer: 2006–2008. The Eighth Report of the Confidential Enquiries into Maternal Deaths in the United Kingdom. *BJOG* 2011; 118 (Suppl. 1): 1–203.

2. Confidential Enquiry into Stillbirths and Deaths in Infancy. *7th Annual Report*. London: Maternal and Child Health Research Consortium, 2000.

3. Confidential Enquiry into Stillbirths and Deaths in Infancy. *5th Annual Report*. London: Maternal and Child Health Research Consortium, 1998.

4. National Maternity Review. *Better Births: Improving Outcomes of Maternity Services in England*. London: NHS England, 2016.

5. NHS England. *Saving Babies' Lives: A Care Bundle for Reducing Stillbirth*. London: NHS England, 2016. www.england.nhs.uk/wp-content/uploads/2016/03/saving-babies-lives-car-bundl .pdf (accessed August 2017).

6. Pehrson C, Sorensen J, Amer-Wahlin I. Evaluation and impact of cardiotocography training programmes: a systematic review. *BJOG* 2011; 118: 926–35.

7. Millde Luthander C, Källen K, Nyström ME, *et al.* Results from the National Perinatal Patient Safety Program in Sweden: the challenge of evaluation. *Acta Obstet Gynecol Scand* 2016; 95: 596–603.

8. Sorensen JL, Thellesen L, Strandbygaard J, *et al.* Development of knowledge tests for multi-disciplinary emergency training: a review and an example. *Acta Anaesthesiol Scand* 2015; 59: 123–33.

9. Thellesen L, Hedegaard M, Bergholt T, et al. Curriculum development for a national cardiotocography education program: a Delphi survey to obtain consensus on learning objectives. *Acta Obstet Gynecol Scand* 2015; 94: 869–77.

10. Draycott T, Crofts J, Ash JP, *et al.* Improving neonatal outcome through practical shoulder dystocia training. *Obstet Gynecol* 2008; 112: 14–20.

11. Weiner CP, Collins L, Bentley S, Dong Y, Satterwhite CL. Multi-professional training for obstetric emergencies in a U.S. hospital over a 7-year interval: an observational study. *J Perinatol* 2016; 36: 19–24.

12. Shoushtarian M, Barnett M, McMahon F, Ferris J. Impact of introducing practical obstetric multi-professional training (PROMPT) into maternity units in Victoria, Australia. *BJOG* 2014; 121: 1710–18.

13. MacRae C, Draycott T. Delivering high reliability in maternity care: in situ simulation as a source of organisational resilience. *Saf Sci* 2016 Nov. https://doi.org/10.1016/j.ssci .2016.10.019 (accessed August 2017).

14. Ayres-de-Campos D, Spong CY, Chandraharan E; FIGO Intrapartum Fetal Monitoring Expert Consensus Panel. FIGO consensus guidelines on intrapartum fetal monitoring: cardiotocography. *Int J Gynaecol Obstet* 2015; 131: 13–24.

15. Lewis D, Downe S; FIGO Intrapartum Fetal Monitoring Expert Consensus Panel. FIGO consensus guidelines on intrapartum fetal monitoring: intermittent auscultation. *Int J Gynaecol Obstet* 2015; 131: 9–12.

16. Visser GH, Ayres-de-Campos D; FIGO Intrapartum Fetal Monitoring Expert Consensus Panel. FIGO Consensus guidelines on intrapartum fetal monitoring: adjunctive technologies. *Int J Gynaecol Obstet* 2015; 131: 25–9.

17. National Institute for Health and Care Excellence. *Intrapartum Care: Care of Healthy Women and Their Babies During Childbirth*. NICE Clinical Guideline CG190. London: NICE, 2014; updated 2017. www.nice.org.uk/guidance/cg190 (accessed August 2017).

Section 10
Pre-eclampsia and eclampsia

Key learning points

- To understand the risk factors for, and recognise the signs and symptoms of, severe pre-eclampsia.
- To understand the potentially dangerous complications of severe hypertension (systolic blood pressure $\geq$ 160 mmHg) and its urgent management.
- To manage an eclamptic fit/seizure effectively.
- To understand the care and monitoring required when a woman is being treated with magnesium sulfate.
- To appreciate the importance of detailed contemporaneous documentation.

Common difficulties observed in training drills

- Not stating the problem clearly when help arrives
- Failing to involve a consultant obstetrician and anaesthetist in the management of women with severe pre-eclampsia and/or eclampsia
- Failure to adequately treat hypertension
- Failure to stabilise the woman, particularly any hypertension, before birth
- Forgetting to perform basic resuscitation during an eclamptic fit/seizure

Aims of the eclampsia scenario

This scenario helps the whole maternity team (midwives, obstetricians, anaesthetists, healthcare support workers, and students) to work through the immediate management of eclampsia, and also demonstrates the teamwork and communication required. There are also additional opportunities for the team to include the differential diagnosis of 'new-onset headache' as highlighted in the 2015 MBRRACE-UK report.[1]

Supporting material

The supporting materials that can be downloaded and printed are:

■ Treatment algorithms for eclampsia and severe hypertension
■ Magnesium sulfate regimen
■ Eclampsia documentation pro forma
■ Partogram of labour progress
■ Maternity notes
■ MOEWS chart

These can all be used in the scenario. There is also an example video which demonstrates the administration of magnesium sulfate. This could be used during the teaching session prior to the drill if it is the same regimen as your local guidelines, but it may be an idea to make your own version to ensure that the regimen and all equipment used are specific to your unit.

Eclampsia scenario

A 40-year-old primiparous woman at 39 weeks' gestation presents to the maternity assessment unit with a severe headache that has not responded to simple analgesia. Her systolic BP is greater than 150 mmHg. The multi-professional team should recognise her hypertension and her potential risk of eclampsia; provide supportive care during the fit and rapidly commence treatment with magnesium sulfate to prevent recurrent seizures; and administer antihypertensive medication to prevent the potential complications of severe hypertension. Once the woman is stabilised, the team is required to make appropriate plans to expedite the birth of her baby.

The team should also consider other causes of sudden-onset severe headache, such as intracranial haemorrhage.

'This is Sophie. She is 40 years old and is 39 weeks pregnant in her first pregnancy. She has had an uncomplicated pregnancy so far. Sophie has presented to the maternity assessment unit with a severe headache that began suddenly 1 hour ago. She has taken paracetamol but unfortunately this hasn't helped the headache. I checked her blood pressure 30 minutes ago and it was 156/94 mmHg. Her booking blood pressure was 120/76 mmHg. Sophie has not yet provided a urine sample. I have just listened to the fetal heart with a Doppler and the rate was 140 bpm.

Sophie, this is [team member's name], she will be looking after you now. I hope you feel better soon. Bye.'

A handover should be given to a member of staff about Sophie (patient-actor). There are several clues in the handover that Sophie may have pre-eclampsia: she has raised blood pressure (both systolic and diastolic) and a 'new-onset headache'. The possibility of pre-eclampsia should be considered by the member of staff taking over Sophie's care. She should re-check Sophie's blood pressure, which will have increased to 160/95 mmHg. This member of staff should also consider continuous fetal monitoring in view of Sophie's raised blood pressure. However, there is no CTG monitoring equipment in the room and she will not have time to go and get it before Sophie has an eclamptic seizure.

After the handover, Sophie (patient-actor) should become increasingly agitated and complain that the light is too bright (photophobia). At approximately 1 minute, Sophie should have an eclamptic seizure. The seizure lasts for approximately 1 minute. Following the seizure, Sophie should remain drowsy and confused for the rest of the scenario.

The team member taking handover should call for appropriate help as soon as Sophie fits, and should also protect Sophie's airway. The team should be able to find, correctly draw up and administer the loading dose of magnesium sulfate as well as simultaneously checking and managing her hypertension, and attempting to monitor the fetal condition. Clearly, the efficient execution of all of these elements will require excellent teamwork and clear instructions from the team leader. Sophie's systolic blood pressure will rise above 160 mmHg during the scenario.

There is no CTG in progress prior to the eclamptic fit, and the team should not rush to commence a CTG or plan for birth until the woman's condition is stabilised with magnesium sulfate to reduce her risk of further fits and her BP has been managed with appropriate antihypertensive treatment, particularly the systolic BP.

The drill should be stopped when Sophie has been stabilised and a plan for birth has been discussed (approximately 8–10 minutes). If a shorter scenario is required, the maternal blood pressure could be kept below 160 mmHg systolic so that blood pressure treatment is not required. For a more complicated scenario, evidence of decreasing oxygen saturations and an increasing respiratory rate could be included, i.e. symptoms of pulmonary oedema.

Equipment

- Patient-actor in night-dress/T-shirt with pregnant uterus (use a towel or cushion)
- Partogram/maternity notes/medication chart
- Sphygmomanometer
- Doppler and CTG machine if available (or use laminated photo of Doppler and cardboard-box CTG machine – see **Appendix 3**)
- Non-rebreather oxygen mask and tubing
- Oxygen saturation machine (or laminated photo)
- Infusion pumps to administer magnesium sulfate (or laminated photo of pump)
- Eclampsia box (clearly marked 'training box' and situated where it would normally be located on labour ward, if possible)
- Simulated version of medication (could be 0.9% saline ampoules re-labelled for vials and sweets for tablets):
  - magnesium sulfate vials
  - labetalol tablets and vials, nifedipine tablets and hydralazine
  - 0.9% saline for dilution
- 1 × 50 mL syringe, 2 × 20 mL syringe, 2 × 10 mL syringe
- Intravenous giving sets
- Cannulae with sharps removed
- Blunt drawing-up needles
- Medication additive labels
- Loading dose and maintenance dose in separate, clearly labelled bags with infusion tubing, drawing up needles, syringes, etc. (Figure 10.1)
- Blood bottles and forms
- Catheter and urometer
- Laminated treatment algorithms and protocols:
  - regimen for administering magnesium sulfate (Figure 10.2)

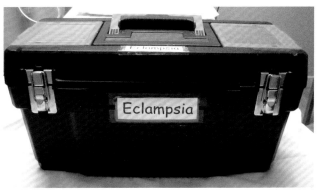
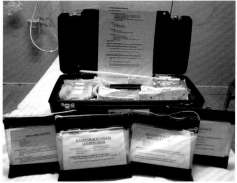

Figure 10.1 Example eclampsia box, including magnesium sulfate
emergency regimen

Loading dose: 4 g magnesium sulfate over 5 minutes

- Draw up 8 mL of 50% magnesium sulfate solution (4 g) followed by 12 mL of 0.9% normal saline into a 20 mL syringe. This will give a total volume of 20 mL.

- Give manually as an intravenous bolus over 5 minutes (4 mL/minute).

Maintenance dose: 1 g/hour

- Draw up 20 mL of 50% magnesium sulfate solution (10 g) followed by 30 mL of 0.9% normal saline into a 50 mL syringe. This will give a total volume of 50 mL.

- Place the syringe into a syringe driver and set the pump to run intravenously at 5 mL/hour.

- Continue infusion for 24 hours following birth or the last seizure, whichever is later.

Recurrent seizures while on magnesium sulfate

- Seek immediate senior help.

- Draw up 4 mL of 50% magnesium sulfate solution (2 g) followed by 6 mL of 0.9% saline into a 10 mL syringe. This will give a total volume of 10 mL.

- Give as an intravenous bolus over 5 minutes (2 mL/minute).

- If possible, take blood for magnesium levels prior to giving the bolus dose.

The maternal condition must be stabilised prior to making plans for birth (if antenatal)

Figure 10.2 Magnesium sulfate regimen

☐ algorithm for managing eclampsia (Figure 10.3)

☐ treatment protocols for severe hypertension (Figures 10.4 and 10.5)

■ Eclampsia documentation pro forma (Figure 10.6)

■ Laminated clinical and teamwork checklists, with pens

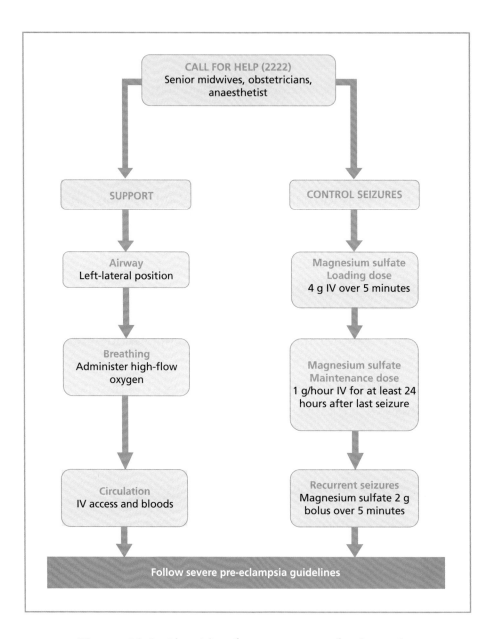

Figure 10.3 Algorithm for treatment of eclampsia

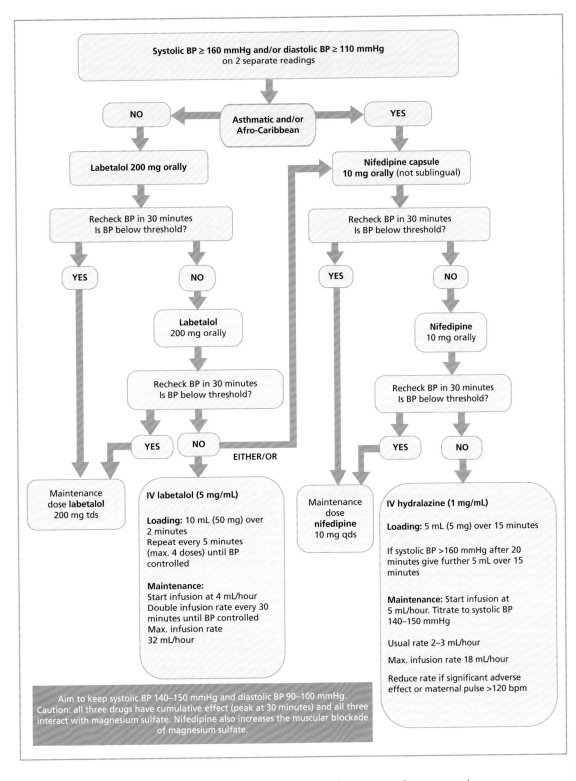

Figure 10.4 Example of algorithm for severe hypertension

Treatment of severe hypertension

- A blood pressure of over 160 mmHg systolic or 110 mmHg diastolic must be treated as a medical emergency
- The aim is to lower the blood pressure to a systolic BP between 140 and 150 and a diastolic between 90 and 100 mmHg. Further reductions do not help the mother and can compromise the fetus
- The maternal blood pressure should be monitored at least every 15 minutes during acute treatment
- The fetal heart should be continually monitored during acute treatment as a sudden drop in blood pressure may cause fetal compromise

Labetalol

■ Ensure the woman is not asthmatic and give 200 mg labatelol orally

■ Recheck the BP at 15 and 30 minutes

■ If the BP has not settled to the target by 30 minutes give a second dose of 200 mg labetalol orally

■ Recheck the BP at 45 and 60 minutes

■ Seek senior advice, if following the second dose of labetalol, the BP still has not settled to the target within 30 minutes. The options for treatment include additional oral nifedipine or IV regimens (labetalol or hydralazine)

Nifedipine

■ If the woman is asthmatic, labetalol is not available and/or has not been effective, give 10 mg nifedipine orally. It is not necessary to give it sublingually, and sublingual administration may cause sudden hypotension and associated fetal compromise

■ Recheck the BP at 15 and 30 minutes

■ If the BP has not settled to the target after 30 minutes, give a second dose of 10 mg nifedipine orally

■ Recheck the BP at 45 and 60 minutes

■ If the BP still has not settled to the target by 30 minutes after the second dose of nifedipine, seek senior advice and change to the IV labetalol or IV hydralazine regimen, dependent on contraindications

Hydralazine

■ If labetalol and/or nifedipine have not been effective or are contraindicated, seek senior help and give IV hydralazine

■ Give 5 mL of 1 mg/mL hydralazine (5 mg) IV over 15 minutes

■ Check the BP at 20 minutes

  ☐ If the systolic is still above 160 mmHg, give a further 5 mL of 1 mg/mL hydralazine (5 mg) IV over 15 minutes

■ If the systolic is below 160 mmHg, start an infusion of 1 mg/mL hydralazine at 5 mL/hr:

  ☐ Titrate the infusion to control the BP

  ☐ The maximum infusion rate is 18 mL/hr

  ☐ The usual infusion rate required is between 2 and 3 mL/hr

  ☐ Reduce/STOP the infusion if the maternal heart rate is above 120 bpm and/or there are any adverse effects

Figure 10.5 Treatment of severe hypertension

Attach Patient ID:

ECLAMPSIA DOCUMENTATION PRO FORMA

DATE: .... TIME OF SEIZURE: .... DURATION OF SEIZURE: ....

PERSONS PRESENT AT ONSET OF SEIZURE...
....

EMERGENCY BELL ACTIVATED   YES / NO   TIME....................................
If emergency bell not activated, please give reason...

	NAME	ALREADY PRESENT (✓)	TIME INFORMED	TIME ARRIVED
EXPERIENCED OBSTETRICIAN				
MIDWIFE COORDINATOR				
ANAESTHETIST				
JUNIOR OBSTETRICIAN				
MATERNITY HEALTHCARE ASSISTANT				
OTHER PERSONS ASSISTING				

CONSULTANT OBSTETRICIAN INFORMED   YES / NO   Name..

If no, give reason...
Time attended (if attended)...

TREATMENT

LEFT-LATERAL POSITION   YES / NO   TIME............................. If no, other position.........................

HIGH FLOW O_2 YES / NO   TIME............................. If no, give reason.............................

IV ACCESS   YES / NO   TIME............................. If no, give reason.............................

BLOODS – GROUP + SAVE   YES / NO   TIME............................. If no, give reason.............................
FBC, CLOTTING, U+Es, LFTs
URATE

MAGNESIUM SULFATE INFUSION (see laminated regimen for dosages)	TIME COMMENCED
LOADING DOSE	
MAINTENANCE DOSE	

INITIAL POST SEIZURE OBSERVATIONS   TIME................................

RESP RATE.................. PULSE RATE.................. BP..................mm/Hg O_2 sats...................% TEMP..................°C

URINARY CATHETER INSERTED   YES / NO   TIME................ If no, give reason......................................

(Commence Maternity Critical Care Chart)

HYPERTENSIVE TREATMENT ADMINISTERED   YES/NO   TIME.......................................
If yes, please document medication given and dosage ....
....

FETAL WELLBEING (if appropriate)   FETAL HEART RATE.................bpm   TIME..............

POST SEIZURE CTG PERFORMED   YES / NO   NORMAL / SUSPICIOUS / PATHOLOGICAL

If CTG not performed, give reason...

Please complete Risk Management Reporting Form and attach copy of this pro forma – Thank you.

Figure 10.6 An example of an eclampsia documentation pro forma

Setting-up instructions

- Ensure that the patient-actor has a pregnant abdomen.
- Ensure that the maternity notes, partogram and MOEWS chart have been printed, and that local fluid and medication charts are available.
- Ensure that all intravenous cannulae have sharps removed.
- Ensure that the eclampsia (training) box is in the correct location and fully stocked. The magnesium sulfate regimen, severe hypertension treatment protocol and eclampsia pro forma should be laminated and placed in the box with a wipe-clean marker tied to the pro forma.

Instructions for drill facilitators

- Hand over to a midwife or doctor in a labour ward room, if possible (the rest of the team should be waiting in an appropriate area outside the room).
- If there is a team observing the drill, they should stand in the corner of the room to observe the scenario; two groups, or individuals, can be allocated to complete the clinical and teamwork checklists.
- Following the handover, the drill facilitator should also stand in the corner of the room. If there is no other team observing, another of the drill facilitators can complete the clinical and teamworking checklists.
- When specific team members are requested to help, the facilitator should go to the door and ask them to attend the emergency. If the emergency call bell is used, all the team members should be asked to attend.
- Generic responses for team members' questions are listed below, under *Laboratory data and bedside tests*.
- The examination findings and laboratory results are listed below and should be made available to the team once the examination has been performed.

Examination findings

- Blood pressure: 175/105 mmHg
- Subsequent blood pressure readings:
  - ☐ if antihypertensive given: 156/98 mmHg
  - ☐ if antihypertensive not given: 176/108 mmHg
- Oxygen saturations: 96% in air
- If a Doppler is used: 'The fetal heart rate is 145 and regular.'

- If a CTG is connected: 'The CTG has a baseline rate of 145 bpm, with normal variability, accelerations present and no decelerations.'
- If a neurological examination is performed: 'There are no focal neurologic signs.'
- If a vaginal examination is performed: 'The cervix is closed.'
- If any other history is requested, give an appropriate response.

Laboratory data and bedside tests

- If blood results are requested: 'Bloods have not been taken yet.'
- If blood has been taken and the results are requested: 'The results are not yet available.'
- If urinalysis is requested: 'Urine has not been tested yet.'

Prompts

Here are some suggestions to facilitate the scenario if the team are struggling to provide the care required:

If magnesium sulfate is not commenced:	'Is there anything that will stop her having another seizure?'
If blood pressure is not treated:	'Is her blood pressure any better yet?'
If fetal monitoring is not commenced after the seizure:	'What is happening to the baby?'
If senior obstetrician/anaesthetist not called:	'Is there anyone else you could call to help her?'

Instructions for patient-actor

- After the handover has finished, the patient-actor should tell the new staff member that: 'My headache is getting worse and my vision is blurry.'
- Following this, answer questions as they are asked in an appropriate manner:
  - ☐ You have been feeling generally unwell for the last two days.
  - ☐ You suddenly developed a severe headache an hour ago.
  - ☐ The pain is mainly in your forehead.
  - ☐ You don't have any visual disturbances or abdominal pain.
  - ☐ You don't usually suffer with migraine or high blood pressure.

- Become increasingly agitated and fidgety and complain that the lights are too bright.
- Approximately 60 seconds after the handover, have a seizure:
  - ☐ Writhe around the bed, moving your legs and arms.
- Stop seizing after about 60 seconds:
  - ☐ Lie, unresponsive, on your back.
- For the rest of the scenario, remain drowsy and just murmur if asked questions.
- Do not have another seizure.

Debrief and feedback

At the end of the scenario, the facilitator could usefully highlight the significance of systolic BP greater than 160 mmHg, and also the differential diagnosis of new-onset headache.

In the UK, the leading cause of maternal death related to pre-eclampsia and eclampsia is intracranial haemorrhage secondary to severe hypertension. Reiterate to participants that the systolic blood pressure is the most important recording and that a systolic blood pressure of above 160 mmHg must be treated as an emergency. Remember to discuss the importance of stabilising the woman prior to planning birth. Explain also that intubation can increase blood pressure, and therefore a woman with significant hypertension should not be given a general anaesthetic until her blood pressure has been controlled.

Emphasise the importance of performing a neurological examination in all women presenting with new-onset headache or headache with atypical features, particularly focal symptoms. The MBRRACE-UK Report identified that the majority of women who died from intracranial haemorrhage presented with a severe headache or sudden collapse, with no previous symptoms.[1] Clinicians should be wary of misdiagnosing these women with migraine.

Finally, highlight the added benefits of magnesium sulfate for neuroprotection of the preterm fetus at 30 weeks' gestation or less, even though the woman in the scenario is at term.

It is important that the management of severe pre-eclampsia and eclampsia is clearly documented. Discuss the use of MOEWS charts for the identification of severely ill women, the use of maternal critical care charts to enable close monitoring of vital signs and fluid input and output, and the use of the eclampsia pro forma to document the management of eclampsia (Figure 10.6).

Following the scenario, the patient-actor may also give feedback to the team on how they thought the team acted in terms of:

Respect:	I felt I was treated with respect
Safety:	I felt safe at all times
Communication:	I felt well informed due to good communication

Eclampsia scenario: clinical checklist

		Time	✓
Call for help	Emergency call bell		
	State the problem		
	Request eclampsia box		
Airway	Turn to left-lateral		
	Maintain airway		
Breathing	Check breathing		
	Administer high-flow oxygen		
Circulation	Insert IV cannula		
	Take baseline bloods		
Displacement	Ensure woman is on left side		
Treatment of eclampsia	4 g bolus of magnesium sulfate (MgSO$_4$) IV over 5 minutes		
	Make up solution correctly		
Maintenance dose	1 g of MgSO$_4$ – correct dose and infusion pump/syringe driver rate		
	Make up solution correctly		
Fluids	If IV fluids administered, use infusion pump (1 mL/kg/h)		
Monitoring	Blood pressure		
	Respirations and oxygen saturation		
	Urinary output		
	Use MOEWS chart or maternal critical care chart		
	Electronic fetal monitoring (after mother stabilised)		
	Vaginal examination (after mother stabilised)		
Treatment of hypertension	Oral/IV labetalol, oral nifedipine or IV hydralazine		
	Aim for target systolic BP of 150 mmHg		
Documentation	Timings of events		
	Medication administered		
	Persons present		

Eclampsia scenario: teamwork checklists

Communication		YES	NO
State the problem	Clinical problem was stated clearly to arriving team		
Instructions	Instructions were clearly worded		
	Unnecessary conversation/noise was avoided		
	Action plans were shared		
	Goals were clearly identified		
Addressed	Specific instructions were given to the appropriate team members		
Sent	Communication was not rushed		
	It was clear what action was required		
Heard	Acknowledgements were made		
	Requests for repeat information were made		
Understood	The information was understood and repeated back by recipient		
	The correct action was performed		

Team roles and leadership		YES	NO
Roles	Each team member had a clear role		
	There was a team leader		
Adaptability	Team members responded well to different situations		
Responsibility	Team members assumed responsibility for their role		
Advocate	Tasks were delegated appropriately		
Feedback	There were regular updates on progress		
	A running commentary was provided		
Support	Team members did not argue about issues		
	None of the team members decided to 'go it alone'		

Situational awareness/standing back, taking a broader view		YES	NO
Notice	There was an awareness of what each member of the team was doing		
	There was an awareness of the resources that were needed		
	Mistakes were identified		
Understand	Regular updates took place throughout the scenario		
	Problems were identified		
	A re-evaluation was undertaken		
	Team members were asked for their opinion		
	Team members were asked to suggest possible solutions		
	A clear action plan was made		
Prioritise	Key tasks were given priority		
Delegate	Each team member had a specific task		
	The tasks were delegated appropriately		

Reference

1. Knight M, Tuffnell D, Kenyon S, *et al.* (eds.); MBRRACE-UK. *Saving Lives, Improving Mothers' Care. Surveillance of maternal deaths in the UK 2011–13 and lessons learned to inform maternity care from the UK and Ireland Confidential Enquiries into Maternal Deaths and Morbidity 2009–13*. Oxford: National Perinatal Epidemiology Unit, University of Oxford, 2015.

Section 11
Maternal sepsis

Key learning points

- Recognise maternal sepsis.
- Importance of using modified obstetric early warning score (MOEWS) charts.
- Importance of senior, multi-professional clinician involvement.
- Use of serum lactate to triage sepsis severity.
- Need for early intravenous antibiotics and fluids.
- Knowledge of the emergency management of sepsis and septic shock.
- Understand the role of the Sepsis Six.
- Awareness that the Sepsis Six is just the initial management, and that ongoing assessment and treatment is also needed.

Common difficulties observed in training drills

- Not stating the problem
- Failure to measure the woman's respiratory rate
- Not plotting clinical observations correctly on a MOEWS chart
- Failure to recognise clinical features of sepsis, especially non-obstetric causes
- Delayed administration of antibiotics
- Failure to treat sepsis with a fluid bolus
- Failure to take microbiology cultures and serum lactate
- Failure to summon appropriate senior support early
- Failure to liaise with critical care if unresponsive to Sepsis Six, or if lactate is greater than 4 mmol/L

Aims of the maternal sepsis scenario

This scenario enables midwives, obstetricians, anaesthetists, healthcare support workers and students to gain experience of the immediate management and teamwork required during a case of maternal sepsis. The team is required to take a history, examine the woman and request the appropriate tests in order to make the diagnosis. Management should include all components of the Sepsis Six administered in the first hour, commencement of maternal critical care monitoring and plans for the birth of the baby.

Supporting material

The supporting materials that can be downloaded and printed off are:

- Maternal sepsis risk assessment tool and Sepsis Six pathway (adapted from UK Sepsis Trust)
- Maternity notes
- MOEWS chart
- SBAR handover sheet
- Blood gas and laboratory blood results

Maternal sepsis scenario

This scenario presents a woman with undiagnosed prolonged rupture of membranes resulting in chorioamnionitis and maternal sepsis. The team should recognise the severity of sepsis by measuring the woman's serum lactate and implement treatment with broad-spectrum intravenous (IV) antibiotics and IV fluids. Once the woman is stabilised, the team is required to liaise with critical care for the ongoing care of the mother, and to make appropriate plans for the birth of the baby.

A handover is given to a member of the participating team about the woman (patient-actor or full-body mannequin, e.g. SimMom). There are several clues in the handover that she may be suffering from sepsis. She has abdominal pain and reduced fetal movements. In addition, she is draining small amounts of greenish offensive smelling liquor. She is also multiparous with a young child (higher risk of group A *Streptococcus* from young child). The possibility of maternal sepsis owing to prolonged ruptured membranes may be considered by the member of staff taking over her care.

'This is Clare. She is 28 years old and is 39 weeks pregnant, in her second pregnancy. She has previously had one normal birth. Clare has arrived in the maternity assessment unit as she is feeling unwell with abdominal pain, which she has had since last night.

She has had no problems in her pregnancy. On arrival, Clare is complaining of abdominal pain, but doesn't think she is having contractions as the pain is constant. She is wearing a pad as she has been draining small amounts of fluid since yesterday, and she also says that the baby has been quieter today.

I haven't done any observations yet, but would you mind taking over and doing these for me, as I have to go to my break now.

Clare, this is [team member's name]. She will be looking after you while I go for my break. Thanks.'

After the handover, Clare (patient-actor) will complain of feeling increasingly unwell with abdominal pain. At approximately 1 minute, Clare has a rigor, complains of feeling very cold and shivery, and asks for extra blankets. Following the rigor, the patient-actor will say that she is frightened at how unwell she is feeling. After this she becomes increasingly drowsy and confused for the rest of the scenario.

Clare's serum lactate (if taken before IV fluid has been given) is 4.5 mmol/L. This serum lactate level reflects the seriousness of the maternal sepsis and should prompt the team to aggressively fluid resuscitate with a fluid bolus of 500 mL crystalloid in 15 minutes (Clare weighs 85 kg), to give intravenous antibiotics, to summon senior help urgently, and to liaise with the critical care team. The maternity team may use the SBAR handover sheet to facilitate the transfer of the clinical information to the critical care team. The fetal heart rate is 160–170 bpm, but the CTG shows normal variability and no decelerations during the scenario, so the team should not be rushing Clare to theatre for an urgent birth, but rather they should be concentrating on stabilising the maternal condition with IV antibiotics and fluid resuscitation before making a plan for birth. Towards the end of the scenario, Clare will also mention that she thinks she is starting to contract. The drill should be stopped when Clare has been stabilised with IV antibiotics and IV fluids, and plans for birth have been discussed (approximately 8–10 minutes).

The team member taking handover would be expected to take Clare's observations and plot them on a MOEWS chart. They should also perform an abdominal palpation, listen to the fetal heart rate, and commence a CTG. They should notice the greenish, offensive fluid on her pad and call for appropriate help. The team should suspect that this is a case of sepsis and use the sepsis risk assessment tool. They should request the sepsis emergency box, and then follow the Sepsis Six pathway, giving high-flow oxygen, securing IV access and sending bloods including a serum lactate (if not already taken), clotting and group and save. They should take blood cultures and a vaginal swab and commence broad-spectrum antibiotics as soon as possible. The choice of antibiotics will depend on local prescribing policies for first-line treatment of severe maternal sepsis. The serum lactate level of 4.5 mmol/L should prompt the team to give a fluid bolus of at least 500 mL of crystalloid in 15 minutes and then re-check the serum lactate after the fluid challenge.

The team should organise for Clare to be transferred to the labour ward and continue to closely monitor her condition, with regular observations, including respiratory rate, plotted on a MOEWS chart or, if available, a maternal critical care chart. Clare should be catheterised and an hourly bag attached so her urine output can be measured and plotted on a fluid balance chart. Once Clare's condition is stabilised, a plan for birth should be made.

Equipment

- Patient-actor in night-dress/T-shirt with pregnant uterus (use a towel or cushion) or a full-body mannequin (e.g. SimMom)
- Maternity notes, MOEWS chart, SBAR handover sheet, local fluid and medication charts
- Thermometer (or laminated photograph)
- Doppler and CTG machine if available (or use laminated photo of Doppler and cardboard-box CTG machine – see Appendix 3)
- Sphygmomanometer and oxygen saturation machine (or laminated photo)
- Maternal sepsis box containing:
  - ☐ laminated maternal sepsis risk assessment tool and Sepsis Six pathway (Figures 11.1 and 11.2)
  - ☐ non-rebreather oxygen mask and tubing
  - ☐ blood bottles and forms (including a blood gas syringe)
  - ☐ blood culture bottles
  - ☐ microbiology swabs
  - ☐ IV cannulae with sharps removed
  - ☐ 2 L crystalloid fluid and IV giving sets

Risk assessment and action for suspected maternal sepsis
(adapted from UK Sepsis Trust Inpatient Maternal Sepsis Tool – 2016)

1. Has MOEWS been triggered?
2. Does the woman look sick?
3. Is the fetal heart rate ≥ 160 bpm?
4. Could this woman have an infection?
   Common infections include:
   - Chorioamnionitis/endometritis
   - Urinary tract infection
   - Wound infection
   - Influenza/pneumonia
   - Mastitis/breast abscess

Affix Patient ID

If YES to any of the above, complete risk assessment

High-risk criteria (tick all those that are appropriate)	Moderate-risk criteria (tick all those that are appropriate)	Low-risk criteria (tick all those that are appropriate)
• Respiratory rate ≥ 25 ☐	• Respiratory rate 21–24 ☐	• Respiratory rates ≤ 20 ☐
• SpO_2 < 92% without O_2 ☐	• Heart rate 100–130 ☐	• Heart rate < 100 ☐
• Heart rate > 130 ☐	• Systolic BP 91–100 ☐	• Systolic BP > 100 ☐
• Systolic BP ≤ 90 ☐	• Temperature < 36°C ☐	• Normal mental status ☐
• Altered mental status/ Responds only to voice, pain or unresponsive ☐	• No urine output for 12–18 hours ☐	• Temperature: 36–37.3°C ☐
• Blood lactate ≥ 2.0* ☐	• Fetal heart > 160 bpm/pathological CTG ☐	• Looks well ☐
• Non-blanching rash/mottled/ cyanotic ☐	• Prolonged ruptured membranes ☐	• Normal CTG ☐
• Urine < 0.5 mL/kg/hr ☐	• Recent invasive procedure ☐	• Normal urine output ☐
• No urine for 18 hours ☐	• Bleeding/wound infection/vaginal discharge/abdominal pain ☐	
	• Close contact with Group A Strep ☐	
	• Relatives concerned about mental/ functional status ☐	
If ONE criterion is present:	• Diabetes/ gestational diabetes/ immunosuppressed ☐	**If ALL criteria are present:**

Commence 'Sepsis Six' NOW	**If TWO criteria are present (also consider if only ONE criterion):**	
• Immediate obstetric review ST3 or higher (transfer to Obstetric Unit if in the community)		**LOW RISK OF SEPSIS**
• Inform consultant obstetrician & consultant anaesthetist	**Send bloods:** FBC, lactate, CRP, U+Es, LFTs, clotting **OBSTETRIC REVIEW (ST3 or higher) within one hour** **Consider 'Sepsis Six'**	**Review and monitor for improvement or deterioration**
• Commence Maternal Critical Care Chart		**Consider obstetric needs and full clinical picture**
• Commence 'High Risk of Maternal Sepsis' pro forma	Review Bloods: If lactate ≥ 2 or acute kidney injury present, follow HIGH risk pathway	

* NB: Lactate measurement may be transiently elevated during and immediately after normal labour and birth. If unsure, repeat sample.

Completed by:
Name: Designation: Time:
Signature: Date:

Figure 11.1 Example of maternal sepsis risk assessment tool (adapted from UK Sepsis Trust[1])

High risk of maternal sepsis pro forma

(adapted from the UK Sepsis Trust

Inpatient Maternal Sepsis Tool – 2016)

Affix Patient ID

CALL FOR HELP and complete ALL 'SEPSIS SIX' ACTIONS within ONE HOUR	Time zero:	
Action	**Time completed & initials**	**Reason not done/ variance/comments**
1. Administer 100% OXYGEN ○ 15 L/min via non-rebreathe mask ○ Aim to keep saturations > 94%		
2. Take BLOOD CULTURES *(but do not delay administering antibiotics)* ○ Also consider sputum/urine/high vaginal swab/throat swab/breast milk sample/wound swab/stool sample, etc.		
3. Take bloods – CHECK SERUM LACTATE ○ If venous lactate raised, recheck with arterial sample ○ Discuss with critical care if lactate ≥ 4 mmol/L ○ Continue to check serial serum lactates to monitor response to treatment (& FBC, CRP, U+Es, LFTs, clotting)		
4. Give IV BROAD SPECTRUM ANTIBIOTICS (as Trust protocol) ○ Administer urgently, consider allergies ○ Aim to take blood culture first but do not delay antibiotics if culture bottles not available		

5. Give IV FLUID THERAPY
 ○ If lactate ≥ 2 mmol/L give 500 mL stat
 ○ If hypotensive or lactate ≥ 4 mmol/L can repeat boluses
  up to 30 mL/kg (e.g. 2 L for a 70 kg woman)
 ○ Extreme caution if woman has pre-eclampsia: discuss
  with anaesthetist		

6. Accurate MEASUREMENT OF URINE OUTPUT ○ Urinary catheter & hourly measurement ○ Document fluid balance record		

If after 'Sepsis Six': systolic BP remains < 90 mmHg, level of consciousness remains altered, respiratory rate > 25, lactate not reducing (or was previously ≥ 4 mmol/L), refer IMMEDIATELY to critical care team

Also consider:
 ○ If antenatal – monitor fetal heart rate/commence CTG
 ○ Remove the source of infection e.g. retained products,
  expedite birth
 ○ Refer to Critical Care Team

Document actions taken:

Maternal sepsis requires multi-professional team input from: (tick staff contacted)

• Midwife coordinator	☐	• Microbiologist	☐
• Senior/consultant obstetrician	☐	• Intensive/critical care team	☐
• Senior obstetric anaesthetist	☐		

Figure 11.2 Example of maternal sepsis documentation pro forma (adapted from UK Sepsis Trust[1])

☐ broad-spectrum IV antibiotics (dependent on local policy) and appropriate fluids, additive labels and drawing-up needles (try to use empty antibiotic vials or normal saline vials re-labelled)

☐ catheter and urometer

■ Laminated blood gas and laboratory blood results

■ Laminated clinical and teamwork checklists, with pens

Setting-up instructions

■ Prior to the scenario, pour some diluted green food dye on to a maternity pad and incontinence sheet to represent offensive, infected liquor.

■ Ensure that the patient-actor has a pregnant abdomen.

■ If using a full-body mannequin, put some pale green stained water into the pelvis to represent infected liquor.

■ Ensure that the maternity notes, MOEWS chart, SBAR handover sheet and the maternal sepsis risk assessment tool and 'Sepsis Six' pathway have been printed, and use local fluid charts etc.

■ Ensure that all IV cannulae have sharps removed.

■ Ensure that the maternal sepsis emergency box (if used in your unit) containing antibiotics, IV fluids, blood culture bottles, swabs and blood-taking equipment is available for the participants to use (Figure 11.3).

■ Ensure that you have laminated copies of the blood results and blood gases so you can hand them to the participants if they perform a blood gas or request blood results.

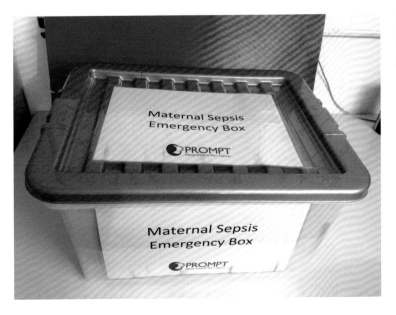

Figure 11.3 Example of maternal sepsis emergency box

Instructions for drill facilitators

■ Hand over to a midwife or doctor in a maternity assessment unit room or labour ward room, if possible (the rest of the team should be waiting in an appropriate area outside the room).

■ If there is a team observing the drill, they should stand in the corner of the room to observe the scenario; two of the team can be allocated to complete the clinical and teamwork checklists.

■ Following the handover, the drill facilitator should also stand in the corner of the room. If there are no other team members free to observe, another of the drill facilitators can complete the clinical and teamworking checklists.

■ As specific team members are requested to help, the facilitator should go to the door and ask them to attend the emergency. If the emergency call bell is used, all the team members should be asked to attend.

■ Some of the responses that may be given if the team members ask for additional information are listed below, under *Laboratory data and bedside tests*.

Examination findings

■ Respiratory rate: 26 respirations per minute

■ Maternal heart rate: 121 bpm

■ Blood pressure: 84/46 mmHg

■ Subsequent blood pressure readings:

☐ if no IV fluids have been given: 76/44 mmHg

☐ if IV fluids have been given: 92/54 mmHg

■ Temperature: 39.2 °C

■ Oxygen saturations:

☐ 93% in air, or

☐ 97% following high-flow oxygen administration

■ Abdominal tenderness, no peritonism

■ Speculum/vaginal examination: green amniotic fluid pooling in vagina

■ Vaginal examination: cervix 4 cm dilated

■ Chest is clear and no other focus of infection evident on examination

■ If a Doppler is used: 'The fetal heart is 155 and regular.'

■ If a CTG is connected: 'The CTG has a baseline rate of 170 bpm, with normal variability and no decelerations.'

■ If any other history is requested, give an appropriate response.

Laboratory data and bedside tests

- If **urinalysis** is requested, the team may be told the following urine 'dipstick' test result:

  - ☐ leucocytes ++

  - ☐ red blood cells negative

  - ☐ nitrites negative

- The **blood result** sheet may be given to the team when requested if they have taken bloods.

- If an **arterial blood gas** sample is taken, give the appropriate results to the team (dependent on whether they have given a bolus of 500 mL of IV fluids).

NOTE: If the laboratory values or reference ranges do not match local protocols, the faculty may wish to prepare a local results sheet that the team will be able to recognise and interpret easily.

- If the team requests **microbiological culture results**, inform them that these are awaited.

Prompts

Below are some suggestions to prompt the team if they are struggling with the scenario:

If maternal deterioration is not appreciated:	'Clare, are you OK?' 'She looks terrible – what's the matter?'
If vaginal examination is not performed (simulated vaginal examination if patient-actor):	'Is Clare's problem anything to do with the green discharge on her pad?'
If no medication is administered:	'Is there anything you can give her for this fever/pain/discharge?'
If senior obstetrician/anaesthetist is not called:	'Is there anyone else you could call to help her?'
If they do not call the critical care team:	'Is there any other specialist you would like to contact to assist with Clare's critical care?'
If the situation is not explained:	'Does Clare understand what's happening?'
If there is no discussion about birth:	'Is the baby OK? Do you want to write a plan for birth?'

Instructions for patient-actor

- After the handover has finished, say: 'I feel really unwell, I have got really bad tummy pain and my baby has been very quiet today, which really isn't like him.'
- Following this, answer questions as they are asked in an appropriate manner:
  - ☐ You have been feeling generally unwell since yesterday.
  - ☐ Abdominal pain today, but it's constant, not like contractions.
  - ☐ Watery vaginal discharge, now turned green colour.
  - ☐ Fetal movements are present, but less than yesterday.
  - ☐ You feel frightened and anxious at how unwell you are feeling.
  - ☐ Towards the end of the drill, mention that you are now having some contractions.
- Negative symptoms/history:
  - ☐ no urinary frequency, urgency, dysuria
  - ☐ no cough/sputum/shortness of breath/chest pain
  - ☐ no headache/neck stiffness/photophobia
  - ☐ no vaginal bleeding noticed
  - ☐ no rashes
  - ☐ no contact history and no travel history
- Become increasingly unwell and agitated, with rapid breathing.
- At approximately 1 minute following the handover, have a rigor:
  - ☐ Start to shiver and make your teeth chatter, complain of feeling really cold and ask for another blanket.
  - ☐ For the rest of the scenario, remain drowsy and respond slowly to any questions.

Debrief and feedback

At the end of the scenario, as part of the debrief, remind participants that sepsis causes a quarter of all the maternal deaths in the UK. Reiterate to participants that early recognition is vital, and that often the patients will express a feeling of 'impending doom' (feel like they are going to die) with life-threatening sepsis. Discuss with them the importance of considering non-obstetric causes of sepsis such as influenza, pneumonia, pyelonephritis and mastitis, which accounted for many of the maternal sepsis deaths in the last Confidential Enquiry, and may be more difficult for obstetricians and midwives to recognise. Discuss that the aim is to provide urgent treatment with broad-spectrum IV antibiotics and IV fluids as per the Sepsis Six in the first hour. Explain that fluids must be given as an initial bolus (comparable to the management of postpartum haemorrhage) and not as a slow maintenance infusion. It is important to emphasise that if a pregnant or postpartum woman does not improve following Sepsis Six management, then this is life-threatening sepsis, and the critical care team should be contacted.

Discuss the importance of serum lactate levels in assessing the severity of sepsis and ensure that all participants know how they can obtain a serum lactate level in their department. Explain that serum lactate levels are elevated during normal labour and birth, and therefore the results from any blood samples taken in this period should be interpreted with caution; if the diagnosis is unclear, then lactate levels should be checked again after birth. Emphasise the importance of involving the critical care team if the lactate is higher than 4 mmol/L, and demonstrate how using the SBAR handover sheet may facilitate the transfer of accurate information to other specialties and members of staff (see Section 4: *Team working and teamwork training*).

This is also a good opportunity to discuss the relevance of a raised temperature as a sign of infection rather than sepsis. In this scenario, Clare had a raised temperature and rigors; however, the typical symptoms of systemic inflammation such as fever may be absent in the most severe cases of sepsis, and in fact hypothermia can be more predictive of the severity of the illness.

Finally, remember to discuss the importance of stabilising the woman prior to birth, and that sepsis may be associated with abnormal clotting. Therefore, this should be checked before a woman is taken to theatre.

It is important that the management of sepsis is clearly documented on the maternal sepsis risk assessment tool and Sepsis Six pathway pro forma. Discuss the use of MOEWS for the identification of severely ill women and the use of maternal critical care charts to enable close monitoring of vital signs and fluid balance.

Following the scenario, the patient-actor may also give feedback to the team on how they thought the team acted in terms of:

Respect: I felt I was treated with respect

Safety: I felt safe at all times

Communication: I felt well informed due to good communication

Sepsis scenario: clinical checklist

		Time	✓
Initial assessment	Take a concise history from woman and perform a full screening examination		
	Perform obstetric and medical examination		
	Complete sepsis risk assessment tool		
Monitoring	Closely monitor respiratory rate, pulse, BP, O_2 saturations, temperature		
	Record observations using a modified obstetric early warning score (MOEWS) chart		
	Abdominal palpation and commence continuous CTG monitoring		
	Transfer to area suitable for maternal critical care		
Sepsis Six	Oxygen therapy via non-rebreather mask		
	Bloods for FBC, U&E, LFT, clotting, **lactate**, random glucose (consider full electrolytes)		
	Microbiology cultures: ▪ Blood ▪ Urine ▪ High vaginal swabs ▪ Throat swab		
	Review and respond to initial results		
	IV broad-spectrum antibiotics		
	IV fluid resuscitation: 500 mL bolus over 15 minutes		
	Catheterise and monitor urine output		
Senior involvement/ critical care	Involve senior obstetrician, anaesthetist, critical care team – SBAR handover sheet		
	Consider microbiological opinion		
	Transfer to labour ward and plan for birth made by team		
Documentation	Document actions on Sepsis Six pro forma		

Sepsis scenario: teamwork checklists

Communication		YES	NO
State the problem	Clinical problem was stated clearly to arriving team		
Instructions	Instructions were clearly worded		
	Unnecessary conversation/noise was avoided		
	Action plans were shared		
	Goals were clearly identified		
Addressed	Specific instructions were given to the appropriate team members		
Sent	Communication was not rushed		
	It was clear what action was required		
Heard	Acknowledgements were made		
	Requests for repeat information were made		
Understood	The information was understood and repeated back by recipient		
	The correct action was performed		

Team roles and leadership		YES	NO
Roles	Each team member had a clear role		
	There was a team leader		
Adaptability	Team members responded well to different situations		
Responsibility	Team members assumed responsibility for their role		
Advocate	Tasks were delegated appropriately		
Feedback	There were regular updates on progress		
	A running commentary was provided		
Support	Team members did not argue about issues		
	None of the team members decided to 'go it alone'		

Situational awareness/standing back, taking a broader view		YES	NO
Notice	There was an awareness of what each member of the team was doing		
	There was an awareness of the resources that were needed		
	Mistakes were identified		
Understand	Regular updates took place throughout the scenario		
	Problems were identified		
	A re-evaluation was undertaken		
	Team members were asked for their opinion		
	Team members were asked to suggest possible solutions		
	A clear action plan was made		
Prioritise	Key tasks were given priority		
Delegate	Each team member had a specific task		
	The tasks were delegated appropriately		

Reference

1. UK Sepsis Trust. Inpatient maternal sepsis tool, 2016. http://sepsistrust.org/wp-content/uploads/2016/07/Inpatient-maternal-NICE-Final-1107-2.pdf (accessed August 2017).

Section 12

Major obstetric haemorrhage

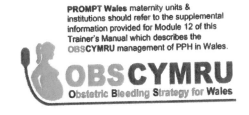

PROMPT Wales maternity units & institutions should refer to the supplemental information provided for Module 12 of this Trainer's Manual which describes the OBSCYMRU management of PPH in Wales.

OBSCYMRU
Obstetric Bleeding Strategy for Wales

Key learning points

- To understand the main risk factors, causes and treatment of major obstetric haemorrhage.

- To consider iron supplementation to optimise haemoglobin concentration before labour and birth.

- To prioritise early fluid resuscitation: intravenous fluid and blood transfusion should not be delayed because of false reassurance from a single haemoglobin result.

- Prompt escalation to senior team members of the multi-professional team.

- For **postpartum haemorrhage (PPH)** – give tranexamic acid (TXA) early (alongside uterotonics).

- Consider the use of cell salvage.

- The importance of 'accurately' measuring blood loss, i.e. weigh blood loss.

- Consider giving blood components before coagulation indices deteriorate.

- Consider early hysterectomy, if medical and surgical interventions are ineffective.

- Document details of management accurately, clearly and legibly.

Common difficulties observed in training drills

- Delay in recognition of the severity of the problem until the woman becomes shocked

- Underestimation of blood loss, and its significance, particularly in smaller women

- Failure to promptly recognise and act on signs and symptoms of haemorrhage

- Delay in commencing adequate fluid resuscitation

- Delay in obtaining senior support and failing to take a 'broader view' of actions required

- Uncertainty of how to access blood products rapidly

- Injudicious use of misoprostol

Major obstetric haemorrhage scenarios

We have included example scenarios for both antepartum (APH) and postpartum haemorrhage (PPH), because although the immediate maternal resuscitation is the same in both cases, subsequent management is very different for antenatal and postnatal women.

Antepartum haemorrhage

Aims of the scenario

This scenario facilitates midwives, obstetricians, anaesthetists, healthcare support workers, student midwives and student doctors to work through the immediate management and the team communication required to manage a woman with a simulated, significant 'revealed' antepartum haemorrhage. There is an emphasis on teaching staff to recognise APH as an emergency and work as a team to manage the APH and expedite the birth of the baby.

Supporting material

The supporting materials that can be downloaded and printed are:

- Treatment algorithm for antepartum haemorrhage
- Modified obstetric early warning score (MOEWS) chart
- Antenatal CTG pro forma and example abnormal CTG
- Poster: Aide memoire for estimating blood loss
- Poster: Example of dry weights to aid more accurate estimation of blood loss

Antepartum haemorrhage scenario

A 22-year-old primiparous woman at 37 weeks' gestation is brought to the labour ward by ambulance with a 30-minute history of continuous abdominal pain and vaginal bleeding.

The multi-professional team should recognise the APH, suspect that there is a placental abruption and declare the emergency, resuscitate the mother and perform a category 1 caesarean section as soon as it is safe to do so.

'This is Sara. She is 22 years old and 37 weeks in her first pregnancy. She is under consultant-led care because she has pregnancy-induced hypertension, a BMI of 18 and anaemia for which she has been taking iron tablets. Her blood pressure has been monitored weekly by her community midwife and Sara has not required any medication, although she was unable to attend her last appointment as she felt unwell.

Sara has been feeling 'tightenings' at home for the past 3 hours but suddenly developed constant sharp abdominal pain 30 minutes ago, and also noticed some vaginal bleeding. The paramedics have estimated 100 mL blood loss so far, but her bleeding appears to be getting heavier.

Sara was very distressed on arrival in the maternity unit, so I have given her Entonox. Her uterus feels tense and it's difficult to tell if she is contracting. I've asked the obstetrician to review her urgently and have commenced a CTG.'

The handover should be provided to a midwife in a labour ward room if possible (if there is no labour ward room free, use another room with the laminated photos of equipment stuck onto walls with Blu-Tack – these are downloadable). This scenario lends itself to having a patient-actor as the woman in labour; also, one of the facilitating team can usefully play Sara's birth partner so that the team can practise their communication in an emergency.

There are several clues in the handover that this woman may be having a placental abruption. Sara has a history of moderately raised blood pressure that had not been taken for almost 2 weeks. She has noticed that her uterus had been tightening at home for 3 hours, before the sudden onset of constant severe abdominal pain, and she also has vaginal bleeding which is initially quite minimal, but is getting heavier on arrival in hospital. The CTG is abnormal from its outset (Sara is not in labour and therefore this would be an abnormal antenatal CTG).

After the handover, Sara (patient-actor) should complain of increasingly severe pain and also of feeling 'light-headed'. She should be increasingly distressed and requesting pain relief. She has one intravenous cannula, sited by the paramedics, but intravenous fluids have not been started. Sara should be lying on the dry, slightly bloodstained (red and blue food colouring) incontinence sheets. She should be told to hold her abdomen (cushion in trousers to simulate pregnant abdomen), and to complain of constant pain and also of feeling vaginal blood loss.

During the drill, a member of staff should take the handover and then call urgently for appropriate help (senior obstetrician, midwife coordinator and anaesthetist). After calling for help, the member of staff should start basic actions including laying the woman on her left side, commencing a CTG to assess fetal wellbeing, administering facial oxygen and preparing for the team to arrive. They may also review the woman's maternity notes, and identify that her placenta was noted to be fundal on the 20-week anomaly scan.

Once the emergency team arrive, it is anticipated that they would quickly introduce themselves, note that the CTG is abnormal (baseline rate 170 bpm, variability less than 5 bpm with unprovoked decelerations), check the vaginal loss, palpate the abdomen and find that the uterus is tense or 'woody' in tone. They should check the 20-week scan for placental siting, and once they have confirmed that it is a fundal placenta they should state that they would perform a vaginal examination. The team should then insert a second large-bore cannula, obtain blood for appropriate tests and contact the laboratory to request cross-matched blood. Resuscitation fluids should be commenced and the theatre team should be mobilised to transfer the woman to theatre for a category 1 caesarean section under appropriate anaesthesia (this may be spinal anaesthesia, or a general anaesthetic may be required if the CTG becomes bradycardic or if the anaesthetist is concerned about coagulopathy). An experienced neonatologist should also be called to attend the birth and given information regarding the abnormal CTG and placental abruption. The team should state that CTG monitoring should be continued until the caesarean section is commenced.

The scenario ends once treatment has been administered to the mother and the theatre team has been summoned for a category 1 caesarean section. For a longer scenario, the team could be asked to manage a PPH following the caesarean section, which is an anticipated problem after an APH, and it could also include neonatal resuscitation.

Equipment

- Patient-actor with a cushion to simulate pregnant uterus
- Magic trousers with material for fake blood
- Fake bloodstained incontinence sheets
- Sphygmomanometer (or laminated photos of local equipment)
- Stethoscope
- Oxygen saturation probe
- Non-rebreather oxygen mask and tubing
- Blood bottles and forms
- Intravenous cannulae (sharps removed)
- Simulated version of medication, labelled 'ranitidine' (could be 0.9% saline ampoules re-labelled)
- Intravenous crystalloid 1000 mL × 2
- Blood giving set × 2
- Gloves
- Catheter and hourly urine bag
- Antepartum haemorrhage treatment algorithm

- Poster: Aide memoire for estimating blood loss
- MOEWS chart
- Cardboard-box CTG machine with CTG attached (see **Appendix 3**) and CTG pro forma
- Local drug and fluid balance charts, consent form
- Laminated clinical and teamwork checklists, with pens

Setting-up instructions

- Prior to the scenario, pour some diluted red food dye (adding in some blue can help with the correct colour) onto an incontinence sheet to represent the vaginal bleeding.

- The patient-actor could be wearing magic trousers with blood material, with a cushion inserted into the waist of the magic trousers to simulate a pregnant uterus; ensure that a small amount of red material is visible before the start of the scenario.

- Sit the patient-actor on the 'bloodstained' incontinence sheet.

- Ensure that all IV cannulae have sharps removed.

- Ensure that the APH treatment algorithm, MOEWS chart, abnormal CTG and antenatal CTG pro forma have been printed, and use local fluid and drug charts etc.

- Ensure that you have laminated copies of the clinical and teamwork checklists available, with pens attached.

Instructions for drill facilitators

- Hand over to a midwife in a labour ward room, if possible (the rest of the team should be waiting in an appropriate area outside the room).

- If there is a team observing the drill, they should stand in the corner of the room to observe the scenario; two groups, or individuals, can be allocated to complete the clinical and teamwork checklists.

- Following the handover, the drill facilitator should also stand in the corner of the room. If there is no other team observing, another of the drill facilitators can complete the clinical and teamwork checklists.

- If possible, another member of the faculty can play the role of the birth partner, to highlight the need for good communication to both the woman in labour and her partner.

- When specific members of the team are requested to help, the facilitator should go to the door and ask them to attend the emergency. If the emergency call bell is used, all team members should be asked to attend.

- If required, the birth partner can help to facilitate the scenario – there are some suitable prompts listed below that may be provided by the birth partner if the emergency team are not taking appropriate action.

- Use the algorithm provided for the initial management of APH (Figure 12.1) to help prompt and guide the team where needed.

Examination findings

- Maternal heart rate: 110 bpm

- Blood pressure: 90/55 mmHg

- Respiratory rate: 18

- Oxygen saturations: 97% in air

- Temperature: 37.0 °C

- Abdominal examination: tense, woody uterus

- Vaginal loss: fresh bleeding

- If a vaginal examination is performed: 'The cervix is 3 cm dilated.'

- CTG: abnormal (170 bpm baseline, with decelerations and reduced variability)

  - ☐ If the team asks about fetal wellbeing, the facilitator should state: 'The CTG is pathological.'

  - ☐ If a plan is not made to perform a category 1 caesarean section, the facilitator can state: 'The CTG is bradycardic.'

  - ☐ If the team attempts to discontinue the CTG to move round to theatre, the facilitator can ask: 'Are you happy to stop the fetal monitoring now?'

- If blood is taken and results are requested, the facilitator should state: 'The results are not yet available.'

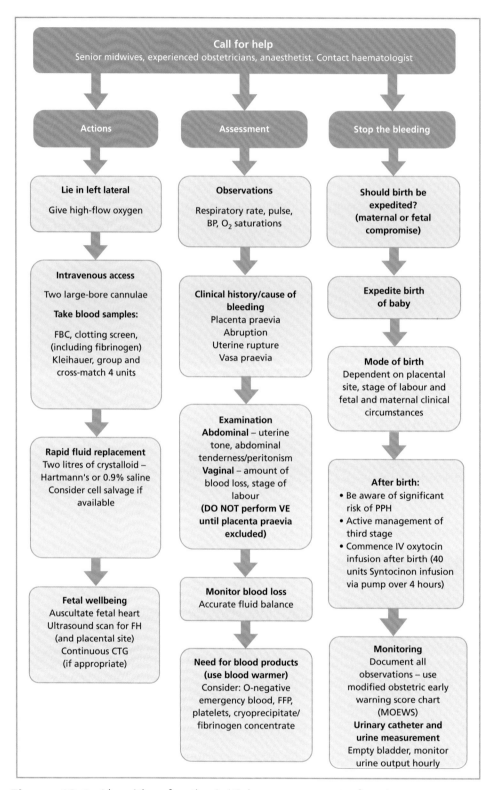

Figure 12.1 Algorithm for the initial management of major antepartum haemorrhage

Prompts

Here are some prompts that the birthing partner can use during the scenario:

Sara is in constant pain, is bleeding heavily and the CTG is abnormal	
If her abdominal pain is ignored:	'Do you think she needs something for the pain?' 'Why is this pain there all the time?'
If the CTG is not addressed:	'Is the baby OK?' 'Is there anything you can do to help the baby?'
If the vaginal bleeding is not acted upon:	'Is this bleeding normal?'
If no decision for caesarean:	'Something is not right – can't she just have a caesarean?
Pain worsening, Sara feeling faint, fetal bradycardia	
If team not responding:	'Something is not right – I'm so worried about the baby. Please can the doctor do something to help them both?' 'I think she is going to faint, she looks so pale'

Instructions for patient-actor

- After the handover has finished, the patient-actor can say: 'I'm in so much pain, it is making me feel light-headed.'
- Following this, answer any questions as they are asked in an appropriate manner, while writhing around in discomfort.
- At approximately 1 minute following the handover, say: 'I'm feeling like I might faint.'
- At intervals throughout the scenario, discreetly pull out a little more red material from the magic trousers.
- If anyone examines or touches your abdomen, complain of severe pain.

Debrief and feedback

At the end of the scenario, the facilitator can usefully discuss the following elements:

- Recognition of placental abruption based upon the clinical history, signs and symptoms.

- Concealed and revealed haemorrhage in cases of placental abruption, and underestimation of blood loss in general. Figure 12.2 is an aide memoire for estimating blood loss that may be printed from the downloadable materials to assist with discussion.

- The importance of the volume of blood loss in relation to the woman's body weight, i.e. women with a lower body weight have a lower circulating blood volume and are therefore less tolerant of blood loss.

- The importance of fluid resuscitation while simultaneously preparing for urgent birth.

- The importance of continuing fetal monitoring until birth.

- Decision regarding category 1 caesarean section.

- Possible choices for anaesthetic, dependent on fetal condition.

Ask the team members marking the clinical and teamwork checklists to give their feedback to the team. The patient-actor and birth partner may also give feedback to the team on how they thought the team acted in terms of:

Respect: I felt I was treated with respect

Safety: I felt safe at all times

Communication: I felt well informed due to good communication

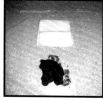

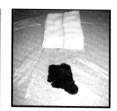

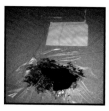

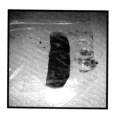

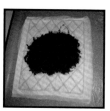

Small swab:
50 mL

Medium swab:
100 mL

Large swab:
350 mL

Sanitary towel:
100 mL

Incontinence sheet:
250 mL

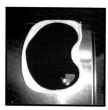

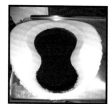

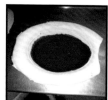

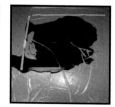

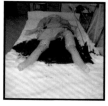

Kidney dish:
600 mL

Bedpan:
500 mL

Vomit bowl:
300 mL

Floor spills:
50 x 50 cm (500 mL)
75 x 75 cm (1000 mL)
100 x 100 cm (1500 mL)

PPH:
On bed only (1000 mL)
Spilling to floor (2000 mL)

Figure 12.2 An aide memoire for estimating blood loss

Antepartum haemorrhage scenario: clinical checklist

		Time	✓
Recognise	Recognise constant abdominal pain		
	Recognise abnormal fetal heart rate pattern		
	Abdominal assessment		
	Vaginal assessment **ONLY** after confirming fundal placenta		
	Recognise risk factors in clinical history		
	Recognise antepartum haemorrhage caused by placental abruption		
Call for help	Summon appropriate help urgently		
	Call for experienced help (including neonatologist once decision made to expedite birth)		
Management	Woman in left-lateral position		
	Administer high-flow facial oxygen		
	IV access and blood for FBC, clotting and cross-match (4 units of blood depending on blood loss)		
	Commence 2 litres IV crystalloid as quickly as possible		
	Decision to expedite birth		
	Plan for category 1 caesarean section		
	Emergency transfer to theatre		
	Decision re appropriate anaesthetic		
	Continuous fetal monitoring until birth		
	Use of MOEWS chart		
Documentation	Timings of events/pro forma		
	Consent		
	Medication administered		
	Persons present		

Antepartum haemorrhage scenario: teamwork checklists

Communication		YES	NO
State the problem	Clinical problem was stated clearly to arriving team		
Instructions	Instructions were clearly worded		
	Unnecessary conversation/noise was avoided		
	Action plans were shared		
	Goals were clearly identified		
Addressed	Specific instructions were given to the appropriate team members		
Sent	Communication was not rushed		
	It was clear what action was required		
Heard	Acknowledgements were made		
	Requests for repeat information were made		
Understood	The information was understood and repeated back by recipient		
	The correct action was performed		

Team roles and leadership		YES	NO
Roles	Each team member had a clear role		
	There was a team leader		
Adaptability	Team members responded well to different situations		
Responsibility	Team members assumed responsibility for their role		
Advocate	Tasks were delegated appropriately		
Feedback	There were regular updates on progress		
	A running commentary was provided		
Support	Team members did not argue about issues		
	None of the team members decided to 'go it alone'		

Situational awareness/standing back, taking a broader view		YES	NO
Notice	There was an awareness of what each member of the team was doing		
	There was an awareness of the resources that were needed		
	Mistakes were identified		
Understand	Regular updates took place throughout the scenario		
	Problems were identified		
	A re-evaluation was undertaken		
	Team members were asked for their opinion		
	Team members were asked to suggest possible solutions		
	A clear action plan was made		
Prioritise	Key tasks were given priority		
Delegate	Each team member had a specific task		
	The tasks were delegated appropriately		

Postpartum haemorrhage

Aims of the scenario

This scenario provides an opportunity for all of the maternity team (midwives, obstetricians, anaesthetists, healthcare support workers and students) to work through the immediate management and team communication required to manage a woman with a simulated postpartum haemorrhage. There is an emphasis on teaching staff to use their local PPH emergency box/trolley and their PPH treatment algorithm, and to work as a team to manage the PPH.

Supporting material

The supporting materials that can be downloaded and printed off are:

- Treatment algorithm for PPH
- Poster: Aide memoire for estimating blood loss
- Poster: Example of dry weights to aid more accurate estimation of blood loss

- MOEWS chart
- PPH documentation pro forma
- Maternity notes

Postpartum haemorrhage scenario

A 40-year-old woman has had a vaginal birth in a birth suite situated next to a consultant-led obstetric unit. She received intramuscular Syntometrine for the third stage of labour. During controlled cord traction of the placenta she starts to bleed heavily and rapidly develops symptoms and signs of hypovolaemia.

The multi-professional team should recognise and declare that there is a PPH. Thereafter, the team should take appropriate steps to administer fluid resuscitation and medication for the treatment of PPH, and, once the woman is stabilised, recognise the need for her urgent transfer to theatre for examination under anaesthesia as there is a suspected retained lobe of placenta. Her subsequent need for maternal critical care should also be considered.

'This is Libby. She is a 40-year-old woman who gave birth to her first baby, Eliza, 10 minutes ago. She had a long labour and pushed for almost 3 hours, so she is very tired but relieved that Eliza is finally born! I gave Syntometrine immediately following the birth and waited a minute before clamping and cutting the cord. During controlled cord traction Libby started to bleed really heavily and the blood has already filled up this kidney dish. The placenta has just delivered but Libby is still bleeding quite heavily. I haven't had a chance to inspect the placenta as yet. The uterus also feels boggy.

Libby, this is [team member's name]. She will be looking after you now as I am going off duty. Congratulations and well done.'

There are several clues in the handover that Libby is at risk of a PPH. She is 40 years old and she has had a long labour. Furthermore, she has already bled significantly as the kidney dish is filled with fresh blood loss and the uterus is atonic. The PPH should be recognised by the member of staff taking over the woman's care.

After the handover, Libby (patient-actor) complains of feeling a bit light-headed and starts yawning and relaxing her hold on her baby. After 1 minute, Libby says she feels faint and then becomes drowsy for the rest of the scenario. These signs (air hunger, fainting and drowsiness) are all features of significant haemorrhage.

Libby should be holding her baby and semi-recumbent on a floor mat. She should be sitting on dry, bloodstained (food colouring) incontinence sheets and wearing the magic trousers with the red material that can be pulled out at regular intervals during the scenario to indicate continuing haemorrhage.

During the drill a member of staff should take the handover and then call for appropriate help (senior obstetrician, midwife coordinator and anaesthetist). After calling for help the member of staff should start basic actions including placing the baby safely in the cot, lying Libby flat on the floor and administering high-flow facial oxygen through a non-rebreather mask.

Once the emergency team arrives, it is anticipated that they would quickly introduce themselves, get the PPH box, gain intravenous access in both arms, take bloods for full blood count, clotting and cross-match, commence 2 litres of crystalloid and administer a second dose of intramuscular/intravenous oxytocin (as Libby has already received one dose for active management of the third stage of labour) and catheterise her bladder. The team should also attempt to expel any clots from the uterus by rubbing the fundus and perform and inspect her perineum and vagina for any significant tears/trauma that could be causing the bleeding. They should also request that someone examines the placenta to check that it is complete.

Despite these initial measures and bimanual compression, Libby continues to bleed, and therefore the team should administer tranexamic acid (TXA) alongside additional uterotonics and consider giving urgent O-negative blood. The scenario will end once Libby is stabilised and the labour ward team have been informed of the need for urgent transfer to theatre for an examination under anaesthetic as there is a retained lobe of placenta.

Equipment

- Patient-actor in a gown wearing magic trousers with red material to be pulled out to indicate bleeding
- 500 mL bag of saline, placed in the front of the magic trousers to represent an atonic uterus
- Baby doll wrapped in towel or blanket

■ Four 'bloodstained' incontinence sheets placed under the patient-actor and on the floor

■ Non-rebreather oxygen mask and tubing

■ Kidney dish (or similar receptacle), coloured dark red

■ **Local PPH emergency box or trolley (**Figure 12.3**) containing:**

☐ PPH emergency treatment protocols

☐ laminated pro forma for documentation

☐ 2 × cannulae with sharps removed

☐ blood bottles and forms

☐ syringes and blunt drawing-up needles

☐ intravenous fluids – crystalloid × 2 L (at least)

☐ 2 × blood giving sets

☐ medication available (could be 0.9% saline ampoules re-labelled):

■ Syntometrine, oxytocin, carboprost (Hemabate)

■ tranexamic acid (TXA)

■ misoprostol (could use small peppermint sweets)

☐ 500 mL normal saline and special giving set for administering oxytocin infusion

☐ catheter and urometer

■ Infusion pumps or laminated photograph

■ Sphygmomanometer/automated blood pressure machine (or laminated photograph)

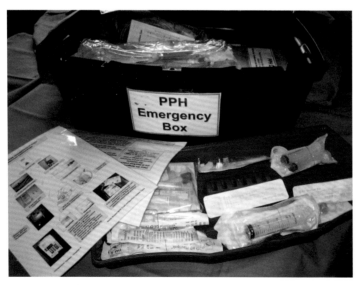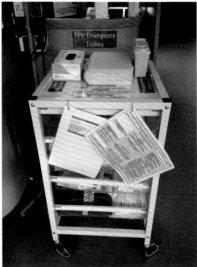

Figure 12.3 Examples of (a) PPH emergency box and (b) PPH emergency trolley

- 2 × laminated photographs of O-negative blood (see **Appendix 3**)
- MOEWS chart
- Poster: Example of dry weights to aid more accurate estimation of blood loss
- Poster: Aide memoire for estimating blood loss
- Maternity notes, fluid chart/drug chart
- Laminated clinical and teamwork checklists, with pens

Setting-up instructions

- Prior to the scenario, pour some diluted red food dye (adding in some blue can help with the correct colour) onto four incontinence sheets and the kidney dish to represent vaginal blood loss.

- The patient-actor should be wearing magic trousers with red material – ensure that some red material is visible before the start of the scenario. Place a 500 mL bag of fluid in the front of the magic trousers to represent an atonic uterus.

- Sit patient-actor on the 'bloodstained' incontinence sheets.

- Ensure that the mother is holding the baby at the start of the drill.

- Ensure that the relevant documentation (as above) has been printed and local fluid and drug charts are available for the team to use.

- Ensure that the drugs required are available in the usual location, i.e. the drug fridge or the PPH emergency box (5 mL vials of saline may be labelled Syntocinon, TXA and carboprost/Hemabate).

- The laminated photographs of the O-negative blood should be placed on top of the blood fridge, as it is important for staff to know the location of the blood fridge and to actually get the 'blood' during the simulated PPH.

Instructions for drill facilitators

- Hand over to a midwife or doctor in a birth suite or labour ward room, if possible (the rest of the team should be waiting in an appropriate area outside the room).

- If there is a team observing the drill, they should stand in the corner of the room to observe the scenario; two of the team members can be allocated to complete the clinical and teamwork checklists.

- Following handover, the drill facilitator should also stand in the corner of the room. If there are no other observers, another drill facilitator can complete the clinical and teamwork checklists.

- When specific members of the team are requested to help, the facilitator should go to the door and ask them to attend the emergency. If the emergency call bell is used, all the team members should be asked to attend.

Time (minutes)	No fluids		1 × IVI Running		2 × IVI running		O-negative blood given	
	Pulse	BP	Pulse	BP	Pulse	BP	Pulse	BP
0 to 3	110	90/60	105	90/60	98	90/60	110	95/65
3+	150	70/40	130	90/60	120	100/60	112	110/70

Examination findings

- Observations: these will depend on the fluid management at that point and are not affected by any medication administered (e.g. oxytocin infusion or Hemabate).
- If an abdominal examination is performed, the facilitator should state that 'The uterus is boggy.'
- If the perineum is inspected, the facilitator should state that 'There is no obvious perineal trauma on initial inspection.'
- If a VE is performed, the facilitator should state that 'There is ongoing bleeding.'
- If the placenta and membranes are inspected, the facilitator can state that 'The membranes are complete but a piece of one of the placental lobes seems to be missing.'

Laboratory requests

The facilitator should respond:

- If blood results are requested: 'Bloods were not taken in labour.'
- If blood has been taken and sent to the laboratory: 'The results are not yet available'
- If cross-matched blood is requested: 'The cross-match will take 40 minutes'
- If type-specific blood is requested: 'Type-specific blood will take 20 minutes'
- If O-negative blood is requested: 'It is kept in the usual place'

Encourage the use of the PPH box and algorithm (Figure 12.4) to prompt and guide the team to provide the best possible care.

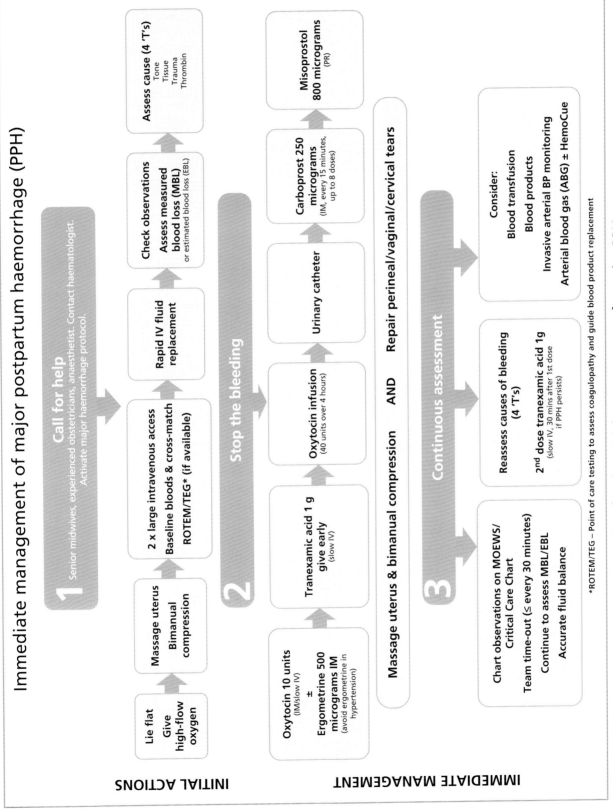

Figure 12.4 Algorithm for the initial management of a major PPH

Instructions for patient-actor

- After the handover has finished say: 'I feel light-headed.'
- Following this, answer any questions as they are asked in an appropriate manner and start yawning.
- At approximately 1 minute following the handover, say: 'I feel faint.' Go floppy and limp and release your hold on the baby.
- For the rest of the scenario you are drowsy and just murmur if asked questions.
- At frequent intervals throughout the scenario, discreetly pull out a length of red material from between your legs.

Debrief and feedback

At the end of the scenario, as part of the debrief, discuss the following:

- The importance of recognising haemorrhage and the significance of maternal tachycardia as a sign of hypovolaemia, even before a fall in the BP.
- The importance of immediate fluid resuscitation.
- The choice of medications administered to treat PPH, and the need to ensure that any clots are expelled from the uterus before commencing a Syntocinon infusion.
- The early use of tranexamic acid (TXA) for treatment of PPH, based on the results of the WOMAN trial.[1] The study results showed a significant reduction in deaths from haemorrhage, and also numbers of laparotomies undertaken to control bleeding, when TXA was given alongside uterotonics, as soon as possible after the onset of primary PPH (and definitely within the first 3 hours), with no adverse side effects. Note that TXA is an antifibrinolytic that prevents the breakdown of fibrin deposits at bleeding sites in the body. It will not produce contraction of the uterine muscle, and should therefore be thought of as an adjunct to the use of uterotonics and surgical control of PPH.
- Use of misoprostol – most useful in low-resource settings (where uterotonics requiring refrigeration are not always available).

- Urgent early transfer to a consultant-led obstetric unit if the woman is at home, or in a midwife-led birth suite.

- Management of PPH if the woman is at home, and the use of bimanual compression as a holding measure while awaiting, and during, transfer.

- That underestimation of blood loss is common and, moreover, the importance of blood loss volume in relation to the woman's body weight – i.e. women with a lower body weight have a lower circulating blood volume and are therefore less able to tolerate blood loss. (You can refer to the aide memoire for estimating blood loss – see Figure 12.2)

It can be useful to facilitate a discussion around the significant and under-reported maternal morbidity following a PPH, and how poor communication and inadequate management of the situation can delay the woman's physical recovery and influence her relationship with her baby and her partner, and her plans for further pregnancies.

Ask the team members marking the clinical and teamwork checklists to give their feedback to the team. Also ask the patient-actor how the team performed in terms of:

Respect:	I felt I was treated with respect
Safety:	I felt safe at all times
Communication:	I felt well informed due to good communication

Documentation

It is important that the management of major obstetric haemorrhage is clearly documented. Discuss the use of MOEWS charts for the early identification of the severely ill woman and the use of the PPH pro forma to document management and treatment. You may also continue the scenario to incorporate the use of the maternal critical care chart.

Postpartum haemorrhage scenario: clinical checklist

		Time	✓
Call for help	Emergency call bell		
	Request PPH box		
Airway	Maintain airway		
Breathing	Check breathing		
	Administer high-flow oxygen using non-rebreather mask		
Circulation	Lie flat or head down		
	Insert 2 large-gauge cannulae		
	Take bloods for FBC, clotting and cross-match 4 units		
Fluids	Commence 2 L of crystalloid		
	Consider O-negative blood		
Treatment	Second dose of oxytocin IV/IM (consider Syntometrine/ ergometrine if not contraindicated)		
	Uterine massage/bimanual compression		
	Empty bladder		
	Oxytocin infusion		
	Tranexamic Acid		
	Intramuscular carboprost (Hemabate)		
	Misoprostol per rectum (if other uterotonics are unavailable)		
	Keep woman warm		
Monitoring	Measure pulse, respiration, oxygen saturations and blood pressure		
	Use MOEWS chart or maternal critical care chart (adapted to include MOEWS)		
	Urinary catheter and hourly measurements		
	Measure blood loss (weigh sheets etc) & provide cumulative blood loss totals		
	Uterine tone		
	Placenta and membranes		
Examination under anaesthesia	Decision once woman is resuscitated		
Documentation	Timings of events		
	Observations and fluid balance		
	Medication administered		
	Persons present		

Postpartum haemorrhage scenario: teamwork checklists

Communication		YES	NO
State the problem	Clinical problem was stated clearly to arriving team		
Instructions	Instructions were clearly worded		
	Unnecessary conversation/noise was avoided		
	Action plans were shared		
	Goals were clearly identified		
Addressed	Specific instructions were given to the appropriate team members		
Sent	Communication was not rushed		
	It was clear what action was required		
Heard	Acknowledgements were made		
	Requests for repeat information were made		
Understood	The information was understood and repeated back by recipient		
	The correct action was performed		

Team roles and leadership		YES	NO
Roles	Each team member had a clear role		
	There was a team leader		
Adaptability	Team members responded well to different situations		
Responsibility	Team members assumed responsibility for their role		
Advocate	Tasks were delegated appropriately		
Feedback	There were regular updates on progress		
	A running commentary was provided		
Support	Team members did not argue about issues		
	None of the team members decided to 'go it alone'		

Situational awareness/standing back, taking a broader view		YES	NO
Notice	There was an awareness of what each member of the team was doing		
	There was an awareness of the resources that were needed		
	Mistakes were identified		
Understand	Regular updates took place throughout the scenario		
	Problems were identified		
	A re-evaluation was undertaken		
	Team members were asked for their opinion		
	Team members were asked to suggest possible solutions		
	A clear action plan was made		
Prioritise	Key tasks were given priority		
Delegate	Each team member had a specific task		
	The tasks were delegated appropriately		

Reference

1.   WOMAN Trial Collaborators. Effect of early tranexamic acid administration on mortality, hysterectomy, and other morbidities in women with post-partum haemorrhage (WOMAN): an international, randomised, double-blind, placebo-controlled trial. *Lancet* 2017; 389: 2105–16.

Section 13
Maternal critical care

Key learning points

- Maternal critical care is required for those pregnant and postnatal women with complex medical and obstetric problems.

- There should be appropriate critical care support for the management of pregnant and postpartum women who become unwell, and this should be provided on the labour ward or a maternal critical care unit.

- Maternal critical care requires the involvement of a multi-professional team of midwives, obstetricians, neonatologists (if mother still pregnant), anaesthetists and intensive care specialists.

- Specialised maternal critical care charts should be used to document observations, fluid balance and ongoing clinical investigations, results and medical reviews.

- Maternal critical care structured review sheets provide a useful framework for structured multi-professional reviews.

- Women requiring maternal critical care should receive frequent obstetric and midwifery reviews to ensure the maintenance of their usual antenatal and postnatal maternity care.

- All carers should be aware of the possible long-term effects of a 'near-miss' incident on a mother's health, in particular her mental health.

Common difficulties observed in training drills

- Incorrect documentation of fluid balance
- Incorrect positioning of arterial line
- Not setting 'goals of the day'
- Failure to optimise the woman's positioning
- Not remembering nutrition/gastric protection
- Not prescribing thromboprophylaxis

Aims of the maternal critical care scenario

This scenario enables midwives, obstetricians, anaesthetists, healthcare support workers and students to gain experience of the immediate postoperative management of a woman requiring critical care. The multi-professional team is required to summarise the intraoperative management, commence a maternal critical care chart and plan her care over the next 4 hours using the maternal critical care structured review sheets as a guide.

The aim of this scenario is for the team to focus on close postoperative monitoring (e.g. correct positioning of the arterial line for blood pressure monitoring, fluid input and output charting, blood investigations and monitoring for signs of further bleeding) and early optimisation of the woman's condition (further blood transfusion, correction of hypothermia, thromboprophylaxis, gastric protection and awareness of pressure areas).

Supporting material

The supporting materials that can be downloaded and printed off are:

- Maternity notes
- Maternal critical care chart
- Maternal critical care structured review sheet
- Blood gas and laboratory blood results

Maternal critical care scenario

This scenario concerns a woman with a BMI of 52 who has just been transferred from theatre following a postpartum haemorrhage (PPH) of 3.4 litres. This was her first pregnancy and she required an operative vaginal birth in theatre for a prolonged second stage. The bleeding appears to be settling, although the mother is tachycardic, hypotensive and hypothermic. The baby weighed 4.6 kg and is well.

'This is Emily. She has just been transferred to the maternal critical care room on the labour ward following a PPH of 3.4 litres in theatre.

This was Emily's first pregnancy. She is 39 years old and had a BMI of 52 at 36 weeks. Her pregnancy was uncomplicated and she went into spontaneous labour at 41 weeks. However, she required an operative vaginal birth in theatre due to a prolonged second stage. Baby Max was born an hour ago; he weighed 4.6 kg and is doing well.

The PPH was due to a combination of atony and vaginal tears. Emily was treated with two doses of IM Syntometrine, one dose of 250 mcg carboprost (Hemabate) IM, 1 g of IV tranexamic acid. A Syntocinon infusion is still running. The vaginal tears have been sutured and the bleeding has now settled.

Emily received one unit (322 mL) of type-specific blood in theatre, together with 2 L of Hartmann's, and 88 mL of a Syntocinon infusion.

She has two large intravenous cannulae and still has her epidural in situ. An arterial line and Foley catheter were sited in theatre. There is 50 mL of concentrated urine in the catheter bag.

Her haemoglobin in labour was 121 g/L. There are three units of red blood cells in the fridge.

Please can you commence her postoperative monitoring and plan her care for the next 4 hours.'

A handover is given to a member of the participating team about Emily (patient-actor or full-body mannequin, e.g. SimMom). There are several clues in the handover that Emily may not have been adequately fluid-replaced in theatre – she is in a negative fluid balance (input = 2410 mL, output = 3450 mL), only 50 mL of concentrated urine has drained and Emily is tachycardic, hypotensive and feeling lightheaded. Furthermore, Emily is hypothermic (a common problem following a massive PPH) and at high risk of venous thromboembolism due to her PPH, obesity and the use of tranexamic acid.

During this workshop the team should recognise:

- The need for close postoperative monitoring (including the use of an arterial line to monitor BP and blood gases, and to take blood).
- The importance of monitoring fluid balance.
- That the mother has not received appropriate fluid resuscitation and requires additional blood transfusion.
- That she is hypothermic and requires warming.
- That she is at high risk of venous thromboembolism and requires thromboprophylaxis.
- That the epidural remains in situ, and its removal should be planned.
- That she is at high risk of developing pressure sores.

The team would be expected to take Emily's observations and plot them on a maternal critical care chart. They should summarise her fluid input and output from theatre on the chart. The team should send a full set of critical care bloods (full blood count, clotting profile, renal function, magnesium, calcium, glucose, liver function, CRP) and also perform a blood gas for immediate assessment of pH, base excess, lactate and haemoglobin to assess the adequacy of the resuscitation thus far. The results that are given to the team later in the scenario – raised lactate (3.1 mmol/L), high negative base excess (–6.3 mmol/L) and low haemoglobin (Hb 79 g/L) – suggest that a further red blood cell transfusion is required.

The team should work through the maternal critical care checklist, which should guide their management of the patient for the next 4 hours.

Equipment

- Patient-actor in a gown with postpartum uterus (use a towel or cushion) or a full-body mannequin (e.g. SimMom) with two large-bore cannulae (one in her right forearm and one in the left antecubital fossa connected to a Syntocinon infusion) and an arterial line in the left radial artery

- Maternity and theatre notes
- Maternal critical care chart, local fluid and medication charts
- Maternal critical care structured review sheet
- Bedside monitor including:
  - ☐ 3-lead ECG
  - ☐ non-invasive blood pressure
  - ☐ oxygen saturations
  - ☐ invasive arterial blood pressure monitoring
- Thermometer (or laminated photograph)
- Forced air warming blanket (or photograph for demonstration)
- Intermittent pneumatic compression devices, e.g. Flowtron (or photograph for demonstration)
- Non-rebreather oxygen mask and tubing
- Blood bottles and forms (including a blood gas syringe)
- IV cannulae with sharps removed
- 2 L crystalloid fluid and IV giving sets
- Three units of red blood cells (laminated photos) in fridge
- Urometer
- Laminated blood gas results
- Laminated clinical and teamwork checklists, with pens

Setting-up instructions

- Ensure that the patient-actor/mannequin has a postpartum abdomen.
- Ensure that the maternity notes, maternal critical care chart and maternal critical care structured review sheet have been printed (use your local hospital charts if you have them), and use local fluid charts etc.

■ Ensure that IV fluids, blood-taking equipment and units of blood (laminated pictures) are available for the participants to use.

■ Ensure that you have laminated copies of the arterial blood gases so you can hand them to the participants if they perform an arterial blood gas.

Instructions for drill facilitators

■ Hand over to a midwife who will be looking after Emily following theatre (it is shift change time). The rest of the team should be waiting in an appropriate area outside the room.

■ If there is a team observing the scenario, they should stand in the corner of the room to observe the scenario; two of the team can be allocated to complete the clinical and teamwork checklists.

■ Following the handover, the drill facilitator should also stand in the corner of the room. If there is no other team observing, a second drill facilitator can complete the clinical and teamworking checklists.

■ As specific team members are requested to help, the facilitator should go to the door and ask them to attend. If the emergency call bell is used, all team members should be asked to attend.

■ Some of the responses that may be given if the team members ask for additional information are listed below.

Examination findings

■ Respiratory rate: 24 per minute

■ Maternal heart rate: 126 bpm

■ Blood pressure: 92/54 mmHg

■ Capillary refill: 4 seconds

■ Temperature: 35.3 °C

■ Oxygen saturations:

☐ 93% on air, or

☐ 97–99% following high-flow oxygen administration

- Chest is clear
- Uterus well contracted, abdomen soft and non-tender
- Normal lochia
- Blood loss in theatre was 3.4 L
- 50 mL concentrated urine in catheter bag
- If any other history is requested, give an appropriate response

Figure 13.1 shows an example of a completed maternal critical care structured review sheet – it gives examples of issues the team should consider when planning management of the woman. You may wish to use this during feedback as a demonstration of a thorough review.

Maternal critical care worksheet		
		Emily Brown *472345*
A	Airway	*Own*
B	Breathing (RR, SpO$_2$, FiO$_2$, chest examination findings)	*RR 24, SpO$_2$ 93% on air/ 99% on 5 litres O$_2$* *Chest clear*
C	Circulation (HR, BP, capillary refill time, requirement for vasopressors)	*HR 126, BP 92/54* *Cap refill 4 seconds, not requiring vasopressor*
D	Deficit (level of consciousness, pain, epidural or spinal block)	*Alert, comfortable, epidural block to T8*
E	Electrolytes (magnesium, sodium, potassium levels and eGFR/creatinine)	*Not measured, need to send urgent bloods*

F	Fluids (input, output, blood loss, drain losses)	*Input: 2410 mL, Output: 3450 mL, 1040 mL negative balance* *EBL: 3.4 L. No apparent ongoing bleeding* *Urine output – only 50 mL concentrated urine in theatre, feels thirsty. ? underfilled*
G	GI & glucose control (bowel function and gastro-protection measures)	*Clear fluids only for next 4 hours* *For gastric protection with ranitidine until on full diet*
H	Haematology (FBC, clotting profile, VTE prophylaxis)	*EBL 3.4 litres, has received 1 unit of RBC, probably needs more blood – for urgent blood gas, FBC and clotting; check RBC units are available* *High risk of VTE but also risk of further bleeding, plus epidural remains in situ therefore for stockings and Flowtrons now. Reassess in 4 hours – ? for LMWH 4 hours after epidural removed*
I	Infection (temperature, inflammatory markers, Sepsis Six, cultures, antibiotics)	*Temperature 35.3 °C* *? septic ? cold from theatre* *For blood cultures, IV antibiotics and serum lactate* *For warming blanket and review in 1 hour*
L	Lines (cannulae, arterial line, central line, urinary catheter, wound drains)	*2 × 16G IV cannulae (right forearm and left antecubital fossa)* *Arterial line in left radial – needs to be zeroed and checked against manual BP* *Foley catheter – change to hourly bag*
O	Obstetric or pregnancy related	*Uterus appears well contracted and minimal blood loss PV, but keep close eye as difficult to assess fundal height with raised BMI*
M	Maternal comorbidities (diabetes, asthma, obesity, epilepsy)	*Emily had raised BMI – 52*
N	Neonatal considerations	*Baby Max – breastfeeding well. Blood sugars being checked regularly*

P	Pharmacology (review drug chart)	*Needs to start IV antibiotics ASAP* *Not for low molecular weight heparin at present, but will need later* *Not for NSAIDs at present due to PPH and poor urine output* *To start oral iron*
Q	Questions	*Is there blood available in the fridge?* *Do we think there is any ongoing blood loss or are we behind on blood replacement?*
R	Recommendations	*For 15-minute observations for first hour and review* *Urgent bloods including arterial blood gas and blood cultures* *Likely to need at least one further unit of RBCs* *Need to start broad-spectrum IV antibiotics ASAP* *To remove epidural catheter as soon as we are confident Emily is unlikely to return to theatre — to review situation in 2 hours* *Warm with forced air warming blanket* *TED stockings and Flowtrons until mobile. Add in LMWH 4 hours after epidural removed*
S	Summary	*3.4 litre PPH, over 1 litre negative balance, poor urine output. Feeling thirsty and lightheaded — for point-of-care testing, haemoglobin assessment and transfusion of at least 1 further unit of RBC* *No signs of ongoing bleeding* *High risk of thromboembolism* *Need to keep warm* *For 15-minute observations plotted on critical care chart* *Change position at least 4-hourly as risk of pressure sores* *Clear fluids only at present with ranitidine gastric protection*
	Signature .... Print .... Date	

Figure 13.1 Maternal critical care worksheet

Point-of-care testing results

The first arterial blood result printout (Figure 13.2) should be given to the team if they take an arterial blood sample.

Towards the end of the scenario you may like to give the team the second set of results which demonstrate clear clinical improvement (Figure 13.3).

NOTE: If the laboratory values or reference ranges do not match local protocol, the faculty may wish to prepare a local results sheet that the team will be able to recognise and interpret easily.

Results			Crit. Low	Reference Low	High	Crit. High
Measured (37.0°C)						
pH	↓ 7.34		[--	7.35	7.45	--]
pCO_2	4.7	kPa	[--	4.6	6.4	--]
pO_2	↑ 22.4	kPa	[--	11.0	14.4	--]
Na^+	133	mmol/L	[--	133	146	--]
K^+	4.6	mmol/L	[--	3.5	5.3	--]
Cl^-	108	mmol/L	[--	95	108	--]
Ca^{++}	1.15	mmol/L	[--	1.15	1.33	--]
Hct	20	%	[--	--	--	--]
Glu	↑ 7.4	mmol/L	[--	3.6	5.3	--]
Lac	↑ 3.1	mmol/L	[--	0.5	2.2	--]
CO-Oximetry						
tHb	79	g/L	[--	--	--	--]
O_2Hb	↑ 98.1	%	[--	95.0	98.0	--]
COHb	1.0	%	[--	--	3.0	--]
MetHb	0.2	%	[--	0.0	1.5	--]
HHb	↓ 0.7	%	[--	2.0	6.0	--]
sO_2	↑ 99.3	%	[--	94.0	98.0	--]
Derived						
BE(B)	-6.3	mmol/L	[--	--	--	--]
AG	11	mmol/L	[--	--	--	--]

Figure 13.2 First arterial blood gas results
The results demonstrate:

- mild acidaemia (pH 7.34)
- metabolic acidosis (BE −6.3 mmol/L, HCO_3^- 18.9 mmol/L)
- raised lactate (3.1 mmol/L)
- anaemia (Hb 79 g/L, haematocrit 20%)
- raised oxygen level as on oxygen therapy (pO_2 22.4 kPa, O_2 saturations 99%)

Results			Crit. Low	Reference Low	Reference High	Crit. High
Measured (37.0°C)						
pH	7.44		[--	7.35	7.45	--]
pCO_2	5.1	kPa	[--	4.6	6.4	--]
pO_2	13.7	kPa	[--	11.0	14.4	--]
Na^+	133	mmol/L	[--	133	146	--]
K^+	3.9	mmol/L	[--	3.5	5.3	--]
Cl^-	105	mmol/L	[--	95	108	--]
Ca^{++}	↓ 1.08	mmol/L	[--	1.15	1.33	--]
Hct	26	%	[--	--	--	--]
Glu	↑ 6.6	mmol/L	[--	3.6	5.3	--]
Lac	↓ 0.4	mmol/L	[--	0.5	2.2	--]
CO-Oximetry						
tHb	99	g/L	[--	--	--	--]
O_2Hb	96.2	%	[--	95.0	98.0	--]
COHb	2.2	%	[--	--	3.0	--]
MetHb	0.7	%	[--	0.0	1.5	--]
HHb	↓ 0.9	%	[--	2.0	6.0	--]
sO_2	↑ 99.1	%	[--	94.0	98.0	--]
Derived						
BE(B)	1.6	mmol/L	[--	--	--	--]
AG	6	mmol/L	[--	--	--	--]

Figure 13.3 Second arterial blood gas results

The results demonstrate:

- normal pH (pH 7.44)
- normal acid/base balance (BE 1.6 mmol/L, HCO_3^- 25.8 mmol/L)
- normal lactate (0.4 mmol/L)
- improving anaemia (Hb 99 g/L, haematocrit 26%)
- normal oxygenation (pO_2 13.7 kPa, O_2 saturations 99%)

Prompts

Below are some suggestions to prompt the team if they are struggling with the scenario:

If maternal critical care chart is not commenced:	'Is there another way of charting her observations and results?'
If maternal critical care structured review sheet is not commenced:	'Do you think a structured review would be helpful?'
If fluid balance is not addressed:	Emily: 'I'm so thirsty, please can I have a drink' or Facilitator: 'Emily, is your urine usually that colour?'

If no blood is administered:	Emily: 'I feel really dizzy and weak. Am I OK?' or Facilitator: 'Oh Emily, you do look very pale. Are you OK?'
If no attempts are made to warm the fluids being given to Emily:	Emily: 'I am really, really cold. Can you turn the heating on?' or Facilitator: 'Gosh Emily, your hands and feet are freezing.'
If the risk of thromboembolism is not discussed:	'Is there anything we need to consider now that Emily will be relatively immobile?'

Instructions for patient-actor

▪ After the handover has finished, say: 'I feel really tired and really thirsty. Can I have a cup of tea please?'

▪ Following this, answer questions as they are asked in an appropriate manner:

  ☐ You feel really cold and want a blanket

  ☐ You feel dizzy and tired

  ☐ You are comfortable and the function of your legs is returning following your epidural top-up

  ☐ Baby Max is well and is going to be bottle-fed by your partner Chris

▪ Negative symptoms/history:v

  ☐ No significant vaginal bleeding

  ☐ No cough/sputum/chest pain/abdominal pain

▪ Become increasingly unwell and lightheaded until a blood transfusion is commenced.

▪ Start to shiver and make your teeth chatter, complain of feeling really cold and ask for another blanket until a warming blanket is used.

Debrief and feedback

At the end of the scenario, as part of the debrief, remind participants that the management of any patient receiving critical care requires a medical review that is comprehensive, structured and regular. A systematic approach should be used involving a 'top-to-toe' examination, together with a regular review of medications, VTE prophylaxis, kidney and bowel function, pain management, fluid balance and nutritional assessment. Regular, structured clinical reviews should ensure that changes in the woman's condition are detected early and timely interventions can be made. Reiterate to participants that early recognition of deterioration is vital, and that often the woman will express a feeling of 'impending doom' (feeling like she is going to die) when suffering from a life-threatening illness. Discuss with them the importance of optimising the condition of the woman by considering all systems, including their psychological state.

Explain the importance of urgent point-of-care testing including pH, base excess, serum lactate and haemoglobin estimation in assessing the severity of the illness and the response to treatment. Explain to participants how to perform these tests urgently within your department.

Emphasise the importance of involving the intensive care team early, and demonstrate how using the SBAR handover sheet may facilitate the transfer of accurate information to other specialties and members of staff (see Section 4: *Team working and teamwork training*).

Following the scenario, the patient-actor may also give feedback to the team on how they thought the team acted in terms of:

Respect:	I felt I was treated with respect
Safety:	I felt safe at all times
Communication:	I felt well informed due to good communication

Documentation

It is important that the management of a critically ill woman is clearly documented and planned on the maternal critical care chart, with 'goals of the day' clearly specified. The maternal critical care chart will also enable close monitoring of vital signs and fluid balance, while the use of a maternal critical care structured review sheet will ensure that a comprehensive multi-professional review and plan of management is made.

Maternal critical care scenario: clinical checklist

		Time	✓
Initial assessment	Take a concise history from woman and handover team		
	Perform an initial top-to-toe medical examination		
	Commence a maternal critical care chart		
Monitoring	Connect to continuous monitoring (3 lead ECG, oxygen saturations, +/- arterial blood pressure monitoring)		
	Closely monitor respiratory rate, pulse, BP, O_2 saturations, temperature		
	Establish hourly urine output monitoring		
	Review blood loss and assess for signs of ongoing bleeding (e.g. uterine height, vaginal loss, peritonism)		
	Record observations on a maternal critical care chart		
Treatment	Oxygen therapy via non-rebreather mask		
	Bloods for FBC, U&E, magnesium, calcium, LFT, clotting, CRP, lactate, random glucose, arterial blood gas		
	Microbiology cultures		
	Review and respond to initial results		
	Transfuse 1 unit red blood cells		
	IV broad-spectrum antibiotics		
	Warm patient		
	Assessment of thromboembolic risk		
Senior involvement/ critical care	Involve senior obstetrician, anaesthetist, intensive care team		
	Thorough review using maternal critical care chart		
	Thorough review using maternal critical care structured review sheet		

Maternal critical care scenario: teamwork checklists

Communication		YES	NO
State the problem	Clinical problem was stated clearly to arriving team		
Instructions	Instructions were clearly worded		
	Unnecessary conversation/noise was avoided		
	Action plans were shared		
	Goals were clearly identified		
Addressed	Specific instructions were given to the appropriate team members		
Sent	Communication was not rushed		
	It was clear what action was required		
Heard	Acknowledgements were made		
	Requests for repeat information were made		
Understood	The information was understood and repeated back by recipient		
	The correct action was performed		

Team roles and leadership		YES	NO
Roles	Each team member had a clear role		
	There was a team leader		
Adaptability	Team members responded well to different situations		
Responsibility	Team members assumed responsibility for their role		
Advocate	Tasks were delegated appropriately		
Feedback	There were regular updates on progress		
	A running commentary was provided		
Support	Team members did not argue about issues		
	None of the team members decided to 'go it alone'		

Situational awareness/standing back, taking a broader view		YES	NO
Notice	There was an awareness of what each member of the team was doing		
	There was an awareness of the resources that were needed		
	Mistakes were identified		
Understand	Regular updates took place throughout the scenario		
	Problems were identified		
	A re-evaluation was undertaken		
	Team members were asked for their opinion		
	Team members were asked to suggest possible solutions		
	A clear action plan was made		
Prioritise	Key tasks were given priority		
Delegate	Each team member had a specific task		
	The tasks were delegated appropriately		

Section 14
Shoulder dystocia

Key learning points

- Understand that shoulder dystocia is unpredictable, and therefore difficult to prevent.

- Understand that during shoulder dystocia, traction should only be applied in an axial direction, using the same force as for a normal birth without shoulder dystocia.

- Be able to perform the manoeuvres required to release the shoulders during shoulder dystocia.

- Understand the importance of clear and accurate documentation.

- Be aware of potential complications of shoulder dystocia, particularly that permanent brachial plexus injury is not inevitable.

Common difficulties observed in training drills

- Not calling the neonatologist
- Failing to state the problem clearly
- Difficulty inserting hand into the sacral hollow
- Confusion over internal rotational manoeuvres, particularly the use of eponyms
- Resorting to excessive traction to release the shoulders
- Using fundal pressure

Aims of shoulder dystocia training

The release manoeuvres for shoulder dystocia are best practised with a mannequin, and this station can be run as a scenario, but should also include practical 'hands-on' training for simulated shoulder dystocia for the entire maternity team (midwives and obstetricians). Student midwives and doctors, paramedics and also accident and emergency staff will also find it useful to practise at least the basic release manoeuvres. There are also important additional elements of the simulation related to the preparation, guidance and communication required to support a woman and her partner during shoulder dystocia.

It is not helpful to use mnemonics or eponyms, because their use has been associated with either no change in brachial plexus injury after training, or even increases in poor outcome. There are also differences in outcomes related to different training mannequins; the PROMPT model was a common theme, together with the use of the RCOG algorithm, in a number of successful training programmes, as is recognised in the RCOG guideline recommendations for training: '*Shoulder dystocia training associated with improvements in clinical management and neonatal outcomes was multi-professional, with manoeuvres demonstrated and practised on a high fidelity mannequin. Teaching used the RCOG algorithm rather than staff being taught mnemonics (e.g. HELPERR) or eponyms (e.g. Rubin's and Woods' screw).*'[1]

There should also be an emphasis on teaching staff to use a specific algorithm of evaluated and effective release manoeuvres. It is equally important that all participants gain hands-on experience of performing these internal manoeuvres during the training sessions.

Supporting material

The downloadable supporting materials include:

- Shoulder dystocia management algorithm
- Maternity notes
- Shoulder dystocia documentation pro forma
- Shoulder dystocia management lecture and demonstration video

There is a PowerPoint lecture and also a video that is particularly useful for the faculty, which demonstrates how a hands-on practical shoulder dystocia workshop should be run, including setting up the PROMPT Flex mannequin

(Limbs & Things, UK), preparing a patient-actor to be the 'mother', and using the algorithm to guide the training session to ensure that all the manoeuvres required for managing shoulder dystocia are demonstrated. You may choose to show some parts of the video to the participants too, either during the lecture (prior to the drill) or at the start of the practical session.

Shoulder dystocia scenarios

There are two example shoulder dystocia scenarios included: the first occurs in the consultant-led maternity unit, and the second scenario in a standalone low-risk birth centre where the shoulder dystocia complicates a pool birth.

Scenario 1: consultant-led maternity unit

A 28-year-old woman in her first pregnancy, who has developed gestational diabetes during her pregnancy, is in spontaneous labour at 39 weeks of gestation and has an epidural in situ for pain relief. She has had a prolonged second stage of labour and, after 65 minutes of pushing, the baby's head is born. However, shoulder dystocia follows and the multi-professional team is required to attend to perform specific manoeuvres to assist with the release of the shoulders.

'This is Kiren. She is having her first baby. She has developed gestational diabetes during this pregnancy and has been diet-controlled. Kiren has laboured spontaneously at 39 weeks. She has an epidural in place and the CTG has been normal throughout labour. Kiren has been pushing for 65 minutes and the baby's head is now born, although there has been some chin retraction. I think she has a shoulder dystocia. Please can you help?'

Scenario 2: standalone midwifery-led birth centre

The second scenario is a 24-year-old woman in her second pregnancy who has had an uncomplicated pregnancy and is now in spontaneous labour at 40 weeks in a standalone low-risk birth suite. She is in the birthing pool and has had a slightly prolonged second stage of labour but, after 40 minutes of pushing, the baby's head is born. There is delay in delivering the shoulders, and therefore the woman is assisted to get out of the pool. Once she is on 'dry land', shoulder dystocia is declared after the next contraction, and the attending midwives are required to perform specific manoeuvres to assist with the release of the shoulders until the paramedic ambulance arrives to transfer mother and baby to hospital.

> 'This is Flora. She is having her second baby. She is now 40 weeks' gestation and has had an uneventful pregnancy. She went into spontaneous labour 4 hours ago and was admitted to the birth centre when she was contracting strongly every 2–3 minutes. On vaginal examination her cervix was found to be 8 cm dilated, so Flora entered the pool. She was confirmed fully dilated 1 hour later and has been pushing for 40 minutes. There has been steady but slow descent of the fetal head. The fetal heart rate has been auscultated intermittently using a Doppler and has been normal throughout labour.
>
> The current situation is that the baby's head is now just crowning, with Flora still in the pool. Please complete the birth.'

Equipment

- Patient-actor to integrate with mannequin, in gown/T-shirt
- Fetal obstetric mannequin such as the PROMPT Flex Birthing Trainer (Limbs & Things, UK)
- MamaNatalie (Laerdal Medical, UK) for Scenario 2
- Towels × 2 for baby and extra towels to dry floor around pool
- Laminated shoulder dystocia algorithm
- Shoulder dystocia documentation pro forma and pens
- Maternity notes

Instructions for drill facilitators

Depending on the experience of the teams undergoing training, you may like to start with a demonstration of each individual manoeuvre on the mannequin before the drill, or demonstrate these afterwards. Either way, it is very helpful to demonstrate the individual manoeuvres during the training session, starting with a view of what shoulder dystocia actually looks like on the mannequin, i.e. the fetal anterior shoulder is impacted on the mother's symphysis pubis – 'bone against bone' – and emphasising that traction will not resolve this problem (Figure 14.1).

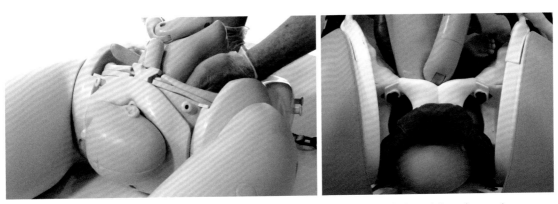

Figure 14.1 Demonstration of the bony problem of shoulder dystocia

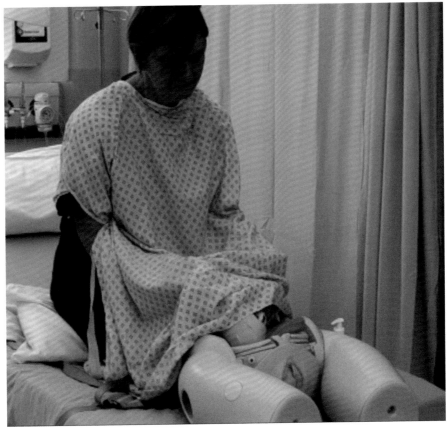

Figure 14.2 Combining a patient-actor with a pelvic mannequin

For Scenario 1, it is useful to integrate a patient-actor and an obstetric mannequin on a labour ward bed (Figure 14.2). The patient-actor should then be advised to maintain the fetal mannequin in shoulder dystocia until the participant has successfully delivered the posterior arm or successfully performed an internal rotational manoeuvre. By using a patient-actor for this scenario the participants can rehearse communication with the mother, which is an essential aspect of shoulder dystocia management. Finally, the participants should document their actions using the shoulder dystocia pro forma. Observers can also complete the shoulder dystocia management clinical checklist for feedback.

For Scenario 2, it is useful for the patient-actor to wear the abdominal part of the MamaNatalie with the PROMPT Flex Baby placed inside it. The patient-actor can then sit in an empty birthing pool (if you have access to a pool room – if not, then pretend that the scenario is starting in the pool). The PROMPT Flex Mannequin can be placed at the side of the pool, and can be used to demonstrate the shoulder dystocia manoeuvres after the scenario has finished.

The participants should ask the woman to leave the pool as soon as they identify delay with the shoulders being born. Once she is out of the pool, the attending midwife should re-check the status of the shoulders, declare the shoulder dystocia and summon appropriate help. They should call for help, including dialling 999 for a paramedic ambulance, and move the woman either on to 'all-fours McRoberts' or flat on her back with her legs in McRoberts' position, and apply suprapubic pressure. Although these simple actions can be effective on their own, in this scenario they will not be; therefore, the midwife participants should move on to attempt to deliver the posterior arm, or perform an internal rotational manoeuvre. Staff who are used to assisting women to give birth in the all-fours position may wish to practise performing internal manoeuvres to resolve the shoulder dystocia with the woman in the all-fours position. It is useful to highlight that in the all-fours position, vaginal access to the sacral hollow will be uppermost.

Instructions for patient-actor

1. After the handover has finished say: 'I want to push.'
2. When help is called into the room ask: 'What is happening?'
3. If you feel that they are not communicating with you, ask: 'Why won't my baby come out?'
4. If you are asked to push, say: 'I'm pushing, I'm pushing!'
5. It is useful to express pain when the manoeuvres are attempted, as they are likely to be painful. Say 'Ow!'
6. Maintain the baby in shoulder dystocia, even though McRoberts' position and suprapubic pressure are performed, until the posterior arm is released or successful internal rotation has been achieved. This will help participants rehearse both the manoeuvres and also the use of the RCOG algorithm (Figure 14.3).

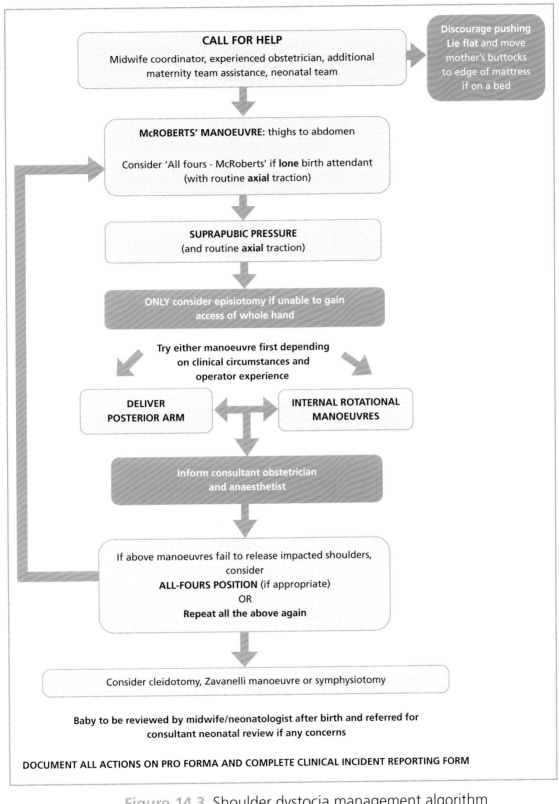

Figure 14.3 Shoulder dystocia management algorithm

Practical training session

During the practical session, it is important that the release manoeuvres are clearly demonstrated, and that there is an opportunity for participants to get 'hands-on' experience. The shoulder dystocia management algorithm (Figure 14.3) should be used during the drills and also for the practical training session, demonstrating each manoeuvre on the mannequin.

Prior to starting the hands-on session, it may be helpful to share an analogy comparing the baby's trapped shoulders to a truck getting stuck under a low bridge (see box).

> ## The truck and the low bridge
>
> A truck passing under a low bridge may be a useful analogy for illustrating shoulder dystocia, and can also be used to explain the anatomical effect of the release manoeuvres:
>
> - The truck drives under a low bridge, which is at a forward-leaning angle. The baby's head is the cab of the truck, and the baby's shoulders and body are the cargo area of the truck. The forward-leaning bridge is the mother's pelvis.
>
> - The baby's head is born – *the cab gets through the bridge* – but the shoulders are obstructed by the mother's pelvis – *the cargo area of the truck gets stuck up against the bridge as the arch of the bridge is too low.*
>
> - Pulling alone will not resolve the shoulder dystocia – *attempting to tow the truck through the bridge once it is trapped, by pulling on the cab, would damage the top of the cargo area and/or the bridge.* The anterior shoulder of the baby is analogous with the top of the truck's cargo area at this point.
>
> - McRoberts' manoeuvre increases the relative diameter of the pelvic inlet and allows space for the anterior shoulder to pass underneath the symphysis pubis – *the forward-leaning bridge becomes upright, making the arch more vertical, thereby increasing the apparent height of the arch of the bridge without changing the actual diameter of the arch, and the cargo area of the truck passes under the bridge.*
>
> - Downward and lateral suprapubic pressure encourages the anterior shoulder into the oblique diameter and then pushes it under the

symphysis pubis, using the relative extra space in the pelvis created by McRoberts' position – *like pressing on the roof of the cargo area so that it slips under the upright bridge.*

- Delivery of the posterior arm makes the baby 10% narrower, so that the anterior shoulder can pass more easily underneath the symphysis pubis – *like taking the wheels off the truck to reduce the height of the cargo area, so that the truck can pass under the upright arch.*

Routine axial traction

It is important to emphasise that routine axial traction (traction that is in line with the axis of the fetal spine) should only be applied to the fetal head to make a diagnosis of shoulder dystocia – 'diagnostic traction' (Figure 14.4). Following this, the only indication for applying the same routine axial traction again is to ascertain whether a manoeuvre has been successful in releasing the shoulders. If the manoeuvre has failed and the shoulder remains impacted, traction should be stopped immediately and the next manoeuvre undertaken.

McRoberts' position

It should also be emphasised that placing a woman in McRoberts' position (thighs against the abdomen) is a simple first manoeuvre that can be very effective (Figure 14.5). The difference between McRoberts'

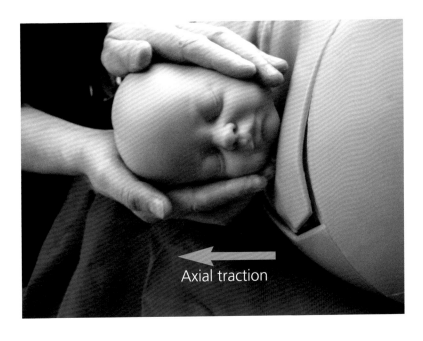

Axial traction

Figure 14.4 Routine axial traction

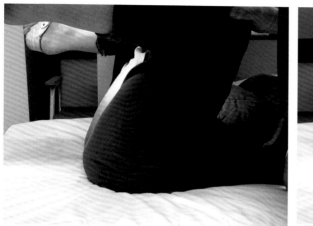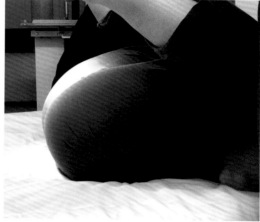

Figure 14.5 McRoberts' position: (a) thighs not sufficiently against the abdomen and therefore buttocks are still resting on the bed; (b) further flexion of maternal hips causes buttocks to lift off the bed, making the pubic arch more vertical

position and lithotomy position should be highlighted. Participants should be reminded that the mother should be laid completely flat with all pillows removed from under her back. A useful indication that McRoberts' has been executed correctly is that the mother's buttocks are lifted off the bed.

Suprapubic pressure

It can be useful to explain that the aims of suprapubic pressure are both to reduce the diameter of the fetal shoulders by adduction and to rotate the shoulders into the wider oblique diameter of the pelvis, to encourage the anterior shoulder to slip underneath the symphysis pubis. Emphasise that an assistant should perform suprapubic pressure from the side of the fetal back where possible, to encourage adduction (narrowing the diameter of the fetal shoulders) (Figure 14.6). If the side of the fetal back is not known, suprapubic pressure can be applied from one side and, if this is unsuccessful, then the other side can be tried.

There is no evidence that suprapubic pressure is better if it is performed continuously, or in a rocking motion. There is also no evidence that suprapubic pressure should be performed for 30 seconds. If the shoulders have not been released by suprapubic pressure, the accoucheur should be encouraged to move on to the next manoeuvre in the algorithm and not resort to applying continual traction to the fetal head. The facilitator should also make sure that participants are not applying pressure directly on the symphysis pubis, but above it.

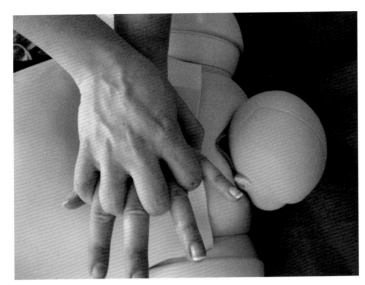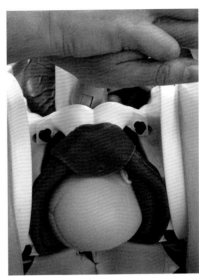

Figure 14.6 Suprapubic pressure

Episiotomy

It is important to stress that an episiotomy will not relieve the bony obstruction of shoulder dystocia and should only be performed to improve access for internal vaginal manoeuvres. There is often enough room for internal access without performing an episiotomy during the shoulder dystocia; often, the perineum has already torn or an episiotomy may have already been performed prior to birth of the head. Therefore, episiotomy should only be considered if there is difficulty gaining vaginal access for the accoucheur's whole hand.

Technique for vaginal access in shoulder dystocia

There can be a temptation to attempt to access the shoulders anteriorly (Figure 14.7a) or laterally (Figure 14.7b), both of which are incorrect. The accoucheur should insert the hand posteriorly at '6 o'clock', into the sacral hollow.

It can be very useful to demonstrate that accoucheurs often attempt to gain access into the vagina as if performing a vaginal examination (Figure 14.7c), with their thumb left outside (Figure 14.7d), thereby making the execution of internal manoeuvres very difficult. The facilitator should explain that inserting the whole hand into the vagina (as if putting on a tight bracelet or reaching for the last Pringle crisp in the bottom of the container) gives the accoucheur more manoeuvrability to attempt either delivery of the posterior arm or internal rotation of the shoulders (Figure 14.8).

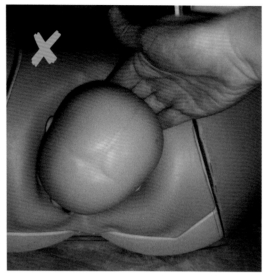

a. Attempting to gain anterior access

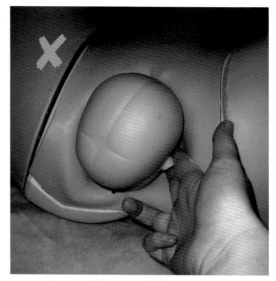

b. Attempting to gain lateral access

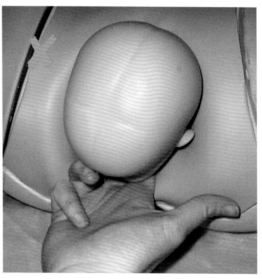

c. Entering the vagina with two
fingers as if performing a routine
vaginal examination

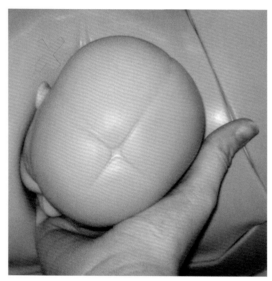

d. Leaving the thumb out of the
vagina

Figure 14.7 Incorrect attempts at gaining vaginal access

Delivery of the posterior arm

Once the whole hand has been inserted into the vagina posteriorly, attempt either to deliver the posterior arm or perform internal rotation. The choice of manoeuvre should depend on the position of the fetal arms and also the accoucheur's experience. It can be helpful to explain (and/or illustrate using a model) that babies tend to lie in the birth canal with their arms flexed across their chest. This means that, as the accoucheur's hand enters the vagina posteriorly, the fetal hand and forearm of the posterior arm may be felt first. If the wrist is then grasped (Figure 14.9a), the posterior arm can be delivered in a straight line (as if raising a hand in class) (Figure 14.9b). Once the

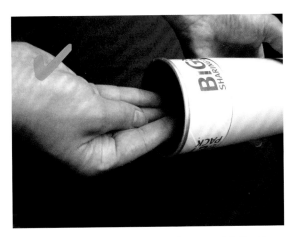
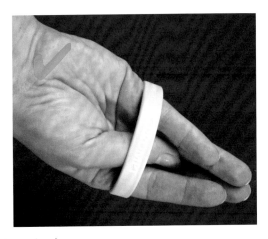

Figure 14.8 Correct vaginal access

(a)

(b)

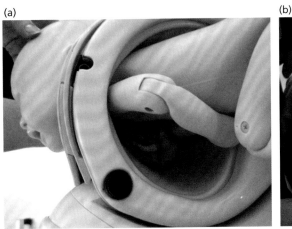
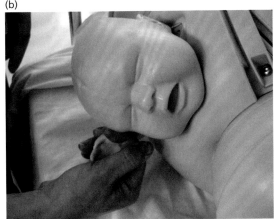

Figure 14.9 Delivery of the posterior arm: (a) grasping the fetal wrist;
(b) the posterior arm delivered in a straight line

posterior arm has been released, routine axial traction can be applied to the fetal head and, if the shoulder dystocia has been resolved, the rest of the baby should be born easily.

In some circumstances it may be very difficult to deliver the posterior arm, as the baby may have a straight arm, or the arm may be behind the fetal chest. In such situations it is usually more appropriate to attempt an internal rotational manoeuvre first, as this is likely to be easier to perform.

If internal rotation is not effective and the baby has a straight arm, do not simply pull on the upper arm. This is likely to result in a fractured humerus. Instead, the fetal arm needs to be flexed to enable the accoucheur to reach the fetal wrist. To flex the fetal arm, pressure should be exerted on the upper arm towards the fetal back. Once the arm has flexed the wrist should be grasped and delivery of the posterior arm should be completed in the manner described above.

Internal rotational manoeuvres

The accoucheur is sometimes reluctant to attempt internal rotational manoeuvres because of confusion between Woods' screw, reverse Woods' screw and Rubin's II manoeuvres. Eponyms should not be used – they cause confusion and the manoeuvres advised today are different to those described originally by Woods and Rubin over 50 years ago.

Internal manoeuvres should be simplified to the concept of trying to rotate the fetal shoulders out of the narrow anterior–posterior diameter and into the wider oblique diameters of the pelvis by applying pressure on the anterior (Figure 14.10a) or posterior (Figure 14.10b) aspect of the posterior shoulder. If rotation is difficult to achieve, internal rotation can be combined with an assistant applying suprapubic pressure in the appropriate direction.

Internal manoeuvres should be documented clearly and descriptively, for example: 'Internal rotation of the fetal shoulders was achieved by pressing on the anterior aspect of the posterior fetal shoulder in a clockwise direction.' Terms such as 'Woods' screw' should not be used.

In addition, discuss alternative and additional management, including consideration of the accoucheur swapping hands to assist birth if they are struggling, or asking another member of the team to attempt internal rotation.

Fundal pressure

Fundal pressure is associated with an increased risk of obstetric brachial plexus injury and also uterine rupture and therefore should not be used.

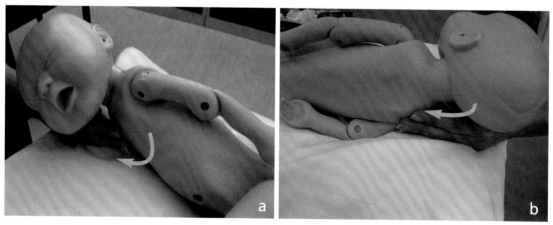

Figure 14.10 Internal rotational manoeuvres: (a) pressure on the anterior aspect of the posterior shoulder to achieve rotation; (b) pressure on the posterior aspect of the posterior shoulder to achieve rotation

Documentation

After a potentially difficult and traumatic birth with a complication such as shoulder dystocia, it is very important that there is clear documentation of the events. It is recommended that a standardised pro forma is used (Figure 14.11).

SHOULDER DYSTOCIA DOCUMENTATION		Mother's Name _____
Date _____ Time _____		Date of birth _____
Person completing form _____		Hospital Number _____
Designation _____		Consultant _____
Signature _____		

Called for help at:		Emergency call via switchboard at:		
Staff present at birth of head:		Additional staff attending for birth of shoulders		
Name	**Role**	**Name**	**Role**	**Time arrived**

Maternal position when shoulder dystocia occurred - please circle (i.e. prior to any procedures to assist)	Semi-recumbent	Lithotomy	Side-lying	All fours	Kneeling	Standing	Squatting	Other ....

Procedures used to assist birth	By whom	Time	Order	Details	Reason if not performed
McRoberts' position					
Suprapubic pressure				From maternal **left** / **right** (circle as appropriate)	
Episiotomy				Enough access / tear present /already performed (circle as appropriate)	
Delivery of posterior arm				**Right** / **left** arm (circle as appropriate)	
Internal rotational manoeuvre					
Description of rotation					
Description of traction	Routine (as for normal vaginal birth)	Other -		Reason if not routine	
Other manoeuvres used					

Mode of birth of head	Spontaneous		Instrumental – vacuum / forceps	
Time of birth of head	Time of birth of baby		Head-to-body birth interval	
Fetal position during dystocia	Head facing maternal **left** / **Left** fetal shoulder anterior		Head facing maternal **right** / **Right** fetal shoulder anterior	
Birth weight ___ kg	Apgar	1 min :	5 mins :	10 mins :
Cord gases	Art pH :	Art BE:	Venous pH :	Venous BE :
Explanation to parents	Yes By ___		Risk incident form completed if clinical concerns	Yes / N/A

Neonatologist called: Yes / No   Time arrived: ....   Neonatologist's name: ....

Baby assessment at birth (maybe done by M/W):			If yes to any of these questions, for review and follow up by Consultant neonatologist
Any sign of arm weakness?	Yes	No	
Any sign of potential bony fracture?	Yes	No	
Baby admitted to Neonatal Intensive Care Unit?	Yes	No	
Assessment by			

Figure 14.11 Example of shoulder dystocia pro forma

Documentation should include the time of birth of the baby's head and body, plus the head-to-body time interval, the direction the baby's head was facing after restitution so that the anterior and posterior shoulders can be clearly identified, the timing and sequence of manoeuvres performed, the condition of the baby at birth (Apgar score and paired cord pH samples), and the staff present during the emergency.

Debrief and feedback

Following the scenario, provide feedback to the team using the clinical checklist and discuss how the manoeuvres were documented. Teamwork checklists are available for printing and can be used for the debrief if running the scenario as a team drill rather than a workshop.

Other useful discussion points at the end of Scenario 2 (the pool birth) could include the importance of getting the woman out of the pool promptly as soon as there is a delay with the birth of the shoulders. It is really important to emphasise that helping the woman out of the pool should not be delayed by trying to attempt manoeuvres in the pool. It is also vital to mention that someone should be allocated to protect the baby's head as the mother steps out of the pool, to ensure that the baby does not spontaneously deliver unaided onto the floor. It is also useful to suggest that they allocate someone to dry the floor once the woman is out of the pool, as staff members, or even the partner, may slip on the wet floor.

Finally, for both scenarios, stress the importance of allocating a member of the team to reassure the mother and her partner, and provide a 'running commentary' of the emergency, as these actions have been demonstrated to help reduce postnatal stress symptoms.

If Scenario 2 has been used, discussion regarding communication with the paramedics and also labour ward staff can be included. In addition, ask the patient-actor to comment on how they thought the team acted towards them in terms of:

Respect:	I felt I was treated with respect
Safety:	I felt safe at all times
Communication:	I felt well informed due to good communication

Shoulder dystocia: clinical checklist

		Time	✓
Call for help	Activate emergency bell		
	Ask for senior obstetrician, senior midwife and neonatologist		
McRoberts' position	Lie woman flat and move buttocks to end of bed		
	Support woman's legs in hyperflexed position – thighs to abdomen (or all-fours McRoberts' if lone birth attendant)		
Suprapubic pressure	Applied correctly and from the side of fetal back		
Routine axial traction	ONLY applies routine traction in an **axial** direction		
Evaluation for episiotomy	Confirm able to gain access of whole hand into sacral hollow		
Delivery of posterior arm	**'Pringles manoeuvre'** – Introduce whole hand into sacral hollow and feel for baby's posterior arm		
	If baby's arms flexed across chest, grasp wrist of posterior arm and deliver arm in straight line (as if putting hand up in class)		
	If baby's posterior arm straight, may be able to flex at the elbow, then grasp wrist and deliver arm in straight line (as if putting hand up in class)		
Internal rotational manoeuvres	**'Pringles manoeuvre'** – Introduce whole hand into sacral hollow		
	Apply pressure to the anterior (front) or posterior (back) aspect of baby's posterior (bottom) shoulder to rotate the shoulders into the oblique diameter		
	If rotation is difficult, ask assistant to apply suprapubic pressure in the appropriate direction		
Inappropriate actions	Excessive force/traction applied to fetal head		
	Traction in downward direction		
	Fundal pressure		
Documentation	Persons present		
	Complete shoulder dystocia documentation pro forma		
	Include: manoeuvres used, head-to-body delivery time, identification of baby's anterior shoulder in relation to mother prior to birth		

References

1. Royal College of Obstetricians and Gynaecologists. *Shoulder Dystocia (Green-top Guideline No. 42)*. London: RCOG, 2012. www.rcog.org.uk/en/guidelines-research-services/guidelines/gtg42 (accessed June 2017)

Further reading

Crofts, J., Lenguerrand, E., Bentham, G. L., et al. Prevention of brachial plexus injury-12 years of shoulder dystocia training: an interrupted time-series study. *BJOG* 2016; 123: 111–18

Section 15
Cord prolapse

Common difficulties observed in training drills

- Difficulties in recognition of occult cord prolapse
- Inappropriate handling of the cord
- Delay in moving the woman to an appropriate position to relieve cord compression
- Not calling for appropriate help
- Difficulties with assembling equipment for bladder filling
- Omitting to take cord gases post-birth

Aims of the cord prolapse scenarios

Two scenarios are presented. They are designed to allow midwives, obstetricians, anaesthetists, healthcare support workers and students to gain experience of the immediate management of a case of cord prolapse, occurring both inside and outside of the hospital setting. Emphasis is placed on teaching staff to recognise the problem and to work as a team to relieve pressure on the prolapsed umbilical cord while taking action to transfer the woman (particularly in the birth-centre setting) and expedite the birth of the baby. In addition, the scenarios reinforce the importance of good communication to the parents and between all members of the multi-professional team.

Supporting material

The supporting materials that can be downloaded and printed are:

- Cord prolapse treatment algorithm
- Maternity notes
- Cord prolapse documentation pro forma
- CTG pro forma
- Blood results

Cord prolapse scenario 1: community setting

During this scenario the team should identify cord prolapse, demonstrate the different methods used to reduce pressure on the prolapsed cord and prepare for transfer to hospital for an urgent assessment. This scenario will highlight some of the potential challenges that may be encountered when an emergency occurs in the community setting, such as transferring the woman from an upstairs room, and also safe positions for transfer of the woman in an ambulance (the woman would not be able to be transferred in the knee–chest position in the ambulance).

Additional factors that the team could consider while waiting for help to arrive include the methods to adopt to relieve pressure on the prolapsed cord, and the appropriate position of the mother, e.g. a knee-to-chest position or exaggerated Sim's (left-lateral with pillow under left hip) (Figure 15.1). Manual elevation of the presenting part may be used to relieve pressure on the cord; however, bladder filling would be preferable as a longer-term measure, as this will facilitate safe transfer of the mother to an ambulance and also free up the midwife to focus on all the other tasks required. Discussions during the debrief session could also include delay or absence of a second midwife arriving at home to help, and the role of the birth partner.

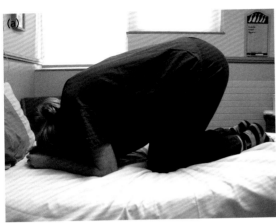
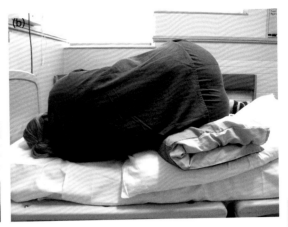

Figure 15.1 Maternal positioning to aid elevation of presenting part:
(a) knee–chest; (b) exaggerated Sim's position

'This is Susan [patient-actor]. She is 30 years old and is 39 weeks pregnant. She has had one previous vaginal birth and has had no problems antenatally. Susan is booked for a home birth and has called you to attend as she is having three contractions every 10 minutes.

Susan's membranes have just ruptured spontaneously with clear liquor draining.'

The patient-actor (Susan) should pretend to be contracting strongly in an upstairs bedroom. Susan's cervix will remain at 5 cm dilated throughout the scenario. The scenario should be conducted following the key points highlighted in the PROMPT *Course Manual*. An important discussion point is the understanding of how the bladder-filling equipment is used, including a demonstration of the procedure. A further point to reinforce is the need to avoid unnecessary delays in transferring the mother, for example by trying to auscultate the fetal heart rate or gaining IV access, which may distract the midwife from performing the vital actions of relieving the pressure on the cord and organising the transfer to hospital. The end point for this scenario will be when the participants have transferred the mother to the ambulance. However, this scenario could also include the necessary actions required once the woman has been transferred into the hospital with learning points incorporated from Scenario 2.

Initial observations

- Maternal pulse: 82 bpm
- Mother: 'I think my waters have gone'

- Blood pressure: 114/80 mmHg
- Respiratory rate: 16
- Temperature: 36.8 °C
- FHR: 134 bpm on auscultation

Cord prolapse scenario 2: hospital setting

During this scenario the team should identify a cord prolapse, demonstrate the different methods used to reduce pressure on the prolapsed cord and prepare for transfer to theatre for an urgent caesarean section. Bladder filling may be considered to elevate the presenting part even if obstetric theatres are nearby, as this could allow enough time for the anaesthetist to administer a spinal anaesthetic prior to this category 1 caesarean section, instead of a general anaesthetic.

The scenario also enables staff to practise transferring a pregnant woman (patient-actor) on a labour ward bed to obstetric theatres in an emergency situation, thus testing their use of local equipment and systems – such as releasing the brakes from the beds, how doors are released to enable beds to pass through, and the passage down narrow corridors. Discussions during the debrief session could also include the RCOG classification of a category 1 caesarean section (immediate threat to life of a woman or fetus) and the difficulty of obtaining informed consent for this procedure in an emergency situation.

> 'This is Betty [patient-actor]. She is 30 years old and is 36 weeks pregnant. She has had one previous vaginal birth and has had no problems antenatally. Betty has come into hospital as she thinks she is in labour. She is now contracting every 2 minutes and they are feeling very strong.
>
> Betty was also seen by her midwife in antenatal clinic yesterday, and she told her that the baby's head was still quite high.'

A CTG is commenced, as Betty is only 36 weeks gestation. The CTG is normal initially, but as Betty mentions that her waters have broken there will be a sudden bradycardia. A section of CTG can be drawn on some CTG paper showing a normal fetal heart tracing and contractions 4:10, with a sudden bradycardia after the membranes rupture. The patient-actor should pretend to have strong contractions and the CTG may be shown to recover once action has been taken to elevate the fetal head off the prolapsed umbilical cord. The cervix will remain at 4 cm dilated throughout the scenario; hence, transfer to theatre for a category 1 caesarean section will be required.

The scenario should be conducted following the actions in the umbilical cord prolapse algorithm (Figure 15.2). The end point should be transfer to theatre on the labour ward bed with the woman in exaggerated Sims' position (left-lateral with pillow under left hip). An operative vaginal birth may be an alternative birth option if the scenario is adapted to be a cord prolapse occurring at full dilatation.

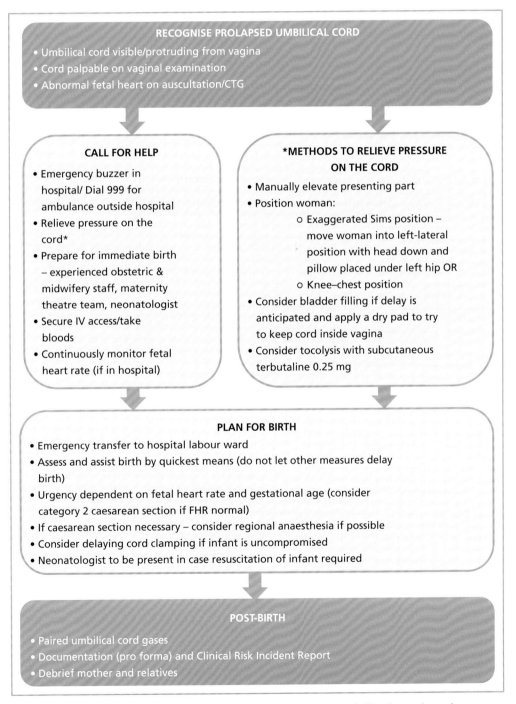

RECOGNISE PROLAPSED UMBILICAL CORD
- Umbilical cord visible/protruding from vagina
- Cord palpable on vaginal examination
- Abnormal fetal heart on auscultation/CTG

CALL FOR HELP
- Emergency buzzer in hospital/ Dial 999 for ambulance outside hospital
- Relieve pressure on the cord*
- Prepare for immediate birth – experienced obstetric & midwifery staff, maternity theatre team, neonatologist
- Secure IV access/take bloods
- Continuously monitor fetal heart rate (if in hospital)

*METHODS TO RELIEVE PRESSURE ON THE CORD
- Manually elevate presenting part
- Position woman:
  o Exaggerated Sims position – move woman into left-lateral position with head down and pillow placed under left hip OR
  o Knee–chest position
- Consider bladder filling if delay is anticipated and apply a dry pad to try to keep cord inside vagina
- Consider tocolysis with subcutaneous terbutaline 0.25 mg

PLAN FOR BIRTH
- Emergency transfer to hospital labour ward
- Assess and assist birth by quickest means (do not let other measures delay birth)
- Urgency dependent on fetal heart rate and gestational age (consider category 2 caesarean section if FHR normal)
- If caesarean section necessary – consider regional anaesthesia if possible
- Consider delaying cord clamping if infant is uncompromised
- Neonatologist to be present in case resuscitation of infant required

POST-BIRTH
- Paired umbilical cord gases
- Documentation (pro forma) and Clinical Risk Incident Report
- Debrief mother and relatives

Figure 15.2 Suggested actions for managing umbilical cord prolapse

Initial observations

- Maternal pulse: 82 bpm
- Mother: 'I think my waters have gone.'
- Blood pressure: 114/80 mmHg
- Respiratory rate: 16
- Temperature: 36.8 °C
- CTG: Sudden bradycardia after spontaneous rupture of membranes occurs

Equipment

- Patient-actor, wearing magic pants with the cushion and baby (see Appendix 3) over the magic trousers (with the red material pushed down the trouser leg, so it is not visible)
- Place pretend placenta (could use the placenta from the PROMPT Flex, or alternatively the magic uterus not inverted but with the cord dangling down) inside the magic pants with the cord protruding out of the vaginal opening of the leg hole of the pants
- For low-risk scenario: handheld Doppler (or laminated photo) or Pinard stethoscope
- For hospital scenario: CTG machine (or cardboard-box CTG machine – see Appendix 3) and hand-drawn trace
- Extra pillow for exaggerated Sims' position
- Cannulae with needles removed
- Blood bottles and forms
- Bladder-filling equipment:
  - ☐ Foley catheter
  - ☐ blood giving set
  - ☐ 500 mL intravenous bag of 0.9% saline to fill bladder
- For hospital scenario: simulated version of medications (could be 0.9% saline ampoules re-labelled):
  - ☐ ranitidine
  - ☐ terbutaline
- Clock for documentation of timings
- Local drug chart and consent forms
- Maternity notes
- Laminated clinical and teamwork checklists and pens

Setting-up instructions

- Ensure that the patient-actor has a pregnant abdomen.

- Ensure that the cord prolapse algorithm, maternity notes and cord prolapse documentation pro forma have been printed and are available for the participating team to use, plus any local medication charts and consent forms.

- Ensure that all intravenous cannulae have sharps removed.

Instructions for drill facilitators

- Hand over to a midwife or doctor in a simulated home setting or a labour ward room (the rest of the team should be waiting in an appropriate area outside the room).

- If there is a team observing the drill, they should stand in the corner of the room to observe the scenario; two of the team can be allocated to complete the clinical and teamwork checklists.

- Following the handover, the drill facilitator should also stand in the corner of the room. If there is no other team observing, another facilitator can complete the clinical and teamwork checklists.

- As specific team members are requested to help, the facilitator should go to the door and ask them to attend the emergency. If the emergency call bell is used in the hospital scenario, all the team members should be asked to attend.

Prompts

Listed below are some questions that may be asked if the team are struggling with the scenario:

If no comment on low fetal heart rate:	'Is the baby ok?'
If vaginal examination not performed:	'Is she in labour?'
If maternal position is not changed, or fetal head not manually elevated, or bladder not filled:	'How could you improve the fetal heart rate?' 'Should you change her position or do something to elevate the presenting part?'
If tocolysis not considered:	'How could you reduce the frequency of the contractions?'
If no plan for birth:	'What are your plans for birth?'

Debrief and feedback

After the scenario, discussion can cover the following:

- The potential challenges faced when a cord prolapse occurs in the community setting.

- Alternative methods of relieving pressure on the cord, e.g. bladder filling, especially when theatre is not immediately available or transfer to hospital is required. It is also useful to check that the equipment that will be used for bladder filling in your unit actually works, and that all connections are water-tight.

- Minimal handling of the cord. There is insufficient evidence to support cord replacement, and no evidence to support the practice of covering the exposed cord with sterile gauze soaked in warm saline. Only a dry pad should be used.

- What actions may be taken if the mother is fully dilated.

- Methods for quickly moving the woman to the ambulance, especially if in an upstairs room at home, i.e. it may be quicker for her to walk downstairs between contractions.

- The importance of communicating with the labour ward coordinator, so that they can prepare for arrival and prioritise workload.

- Communication of the urgency of the caesarean section to the team (in hospital setting).

- Issues of consent in an emergency:
  - validity of written versus verbal consent in an emergency
  - standardised consent form for caesarean section
  - further discussion available from the RCOG Consent Advice document.[1]

- It is worth emphasising that there is good evidence to suggest that the time interval between decision and birth can be significantly reduced by getting the whole team to practise the 38 potential actions required when a cord prolapse occurs.[2]

- The importance of debriefing the mother, partner and staff involved after the event.

The patient-actor may give feedback about how they thought the team acted in terms of:

Respect:	I felt I was treated with respect
Safety:	I felt safe at all times
Communication:	I felt well informed due to good communication

Documentation

All actions, manoeuvres and timings should be documented clearly.
Figure 15.3 is an example of a pro forma that could be used.

Cord prolapse scenario: clinical checklist

		Time	✔
Recognise	Recognise abnormal fetal heart rate (may not always be abnormal)		
	Vaginal assessment		
	Diagnose cord prolapse		
Call for help	Emergency bell/call for ambulance/second midwife		
	Call for experienced help (including neonatologist) (if hospital setting)		
Relieve pressure on cord	Woman in exaggerated Sims'/knee–chest position		
	Manually elevate presenting part		
	Consider bladder filling		
	Consider tocolysis (if hospital)		
Plan for birth	Emergency transfer to theatre/hospital		
	Plan for appropriate method of birth (if hospital setting): ▪ Monitor fetal heart rate ▪ IV access and take bloods ▪ Category 1 caesarean section ▪ Operative vaginal birth		
Documentation	Consent		
	Timings of events/pro forma		
	Medication administered (if hospital)		
	Persons present		

CORD PROLAPSE PROFORMA

	Addressograph
	or name and unit no

Please tick the relevant boxes

Diagnosed: **Home** ☐   **Birth Centre** ☐   **CDS** ☐   **Ward** ☐

Time of diagnosis:...........................

Cervical dilatation at diagnosis: .... cm

If at Home / Birth Centre

Ambulance called?   Yes ☐ No ☐   **Time called:** ....   **Arrived:** ....

CDS contacted?   Yes ☐ No☐   **Time called:** ....   **Arrival time at Hospital:** ....

If on CDS/Ward

Senior Midwife called   **Yes** ☐   **No** ☐   Time............   Arrived.................

Senior Obstetrician called   **Yes** ☐   **No** ☐   Time............   Arrived.................

Grade of Obstetrician: ....

Neonatologist called   **Yes** ☐   **No** ☐   Time............   Arrived.................

Procedure used in managing cord prolapse				
Elevating the presenting part manually	**Yes** ☐		**No** ☐	
Filling the bladder	**Yes** ☐		**No** ☐	
Exaggerated Sims (left lateral) / Knee-Chest position / Head Tilt / Trolley / Bed **(Please circle)**				
Tocolysis with sc Terbutaline 0.25 mg or other	**Yes** ☐		**No** ☐	
Decision to birth interval: ....minutes				

Mode of birth		Mode of Anaesthesia	
Spontaneous vaginal	☐	GA	☐
Forceps	☐	Spinal	☐
Ventouse	☐	Epidural	☐
LSCS	☐		

Apgar Score		Baby's weight:	
:1 min		Cord pH	Base Excess:
:5 min		Venous:	
:10 min		Arterial:	
Admission to NICU? **Yes** ☐ **No** ☐			
Clinical Incident Reporting form completed? **Yes** ☐			
Known Risk Factor? **YES** ☐ **NO** ☐ If YES, please state:			
Mother debriefed **Yes** ☐ **No** ☐			

Signature: ....   Print: ....

Designation: ....   Date: ....

Figure 15.3 An example of a cord prolapse documentation pro forma

Cord prolapse scenario: teamwork checklists

Communication		YES	NO
State the problem	Clinical problem was stated clearly to arriving team		
Instructions	Instructions were clearly worded		
	Unnecessary conversation/noise was avoided		
	Action plans were shared		
	Goals were clearly identified		
Addressed	Specific instructions were given to the appropriate team members		
Sent	Communication was not rushed		
	It was clear what action was required		
Heard	Acknowledgements were made		
	Requests for repeat information were made		
Understood	The information was understood and repeated back by recipient		
	The correct action was performed		

Team roles and leadership		YES	NO
Roles	Each team member had a clear role		
	There was a team leader		
Adaptability	Team members responded well to different situations		
Responsibility	Team members assumed responsibility for their role		
Advocate	Tasks were delegated appropriately		
Feedback	There were regular updates on progress		
	A running commentary was provided		
Support	Team members did not argue about issues		
	None of the team members decided to 'go it alone'		

Situational awareness/standing back, taking a broader view		YES	NO
Notice	There was an awareness of what each member of the team was doing		
	There was an awareness of the resources that were needed		
	Mistakes were identified		
Understand	Regular updates took place throughout the scenario		
	Problems were identified		
	A re-evaluation was undertaken		
	Team members were asked for their opinion		
	Team members were asked to suggest possible solutions		
	A clear action plan was made		
Prioritise	Key tasks were given priority		
Delegate	Each team member had a specific task		
	The tasks were delegated appropriately		

References

1. Royal College of Obstetricians and Gynaecologists. *Caesarean Section*, 2nd edn. Consent Advice No. 7. London: RCOG, 2009. https://www.rcog.org.uk/en/guidelines-research-services/guidelines/consent-advice-7 (accessed August 2017).

2. Siassakos D, Hasafa Z, Sibanda T, *et al.* Retrospective cohort study of diagnosis–delivery interval with umbilical cord prolapse: the effect of team training. *BJOG* 2009; 116: 1089–96.

Section 16
Vaginal breech birth

Key learning points

- Ensure that practitioners managing vaginal breech birth are trained and competent.
- Ensure that there is continuous electronic fetal monitoring during labour and birth (even if the decision is taken to perform a caesarean section), as this may lead to improved neonatal outcomes.
- Ensure full cervical dilatation before commencing pushing.
- Await visualisation of the breech at the perineum before encouraging active pushing.
- Avoid traction on the breech.
- Ensure a 'hands off' approach as much as possible.
- Understand the manoeuvres that may be required to assist a vaginal breech birth.

Common difficulties observed in training drills

- Reluctance to allow the breech to descend without intervention
- Premature commencement of assisted breech manoeuvres
- Pressure on the infant's abdomen away from bony prominences during those manoeuvres
- Failing to flex knees and elbows in the correct direction during release manoeuvres
- Overextending the neck during birth of the head

Aims of the breech birth scenario

Whether it is run as a practical training session or as a simulated emergency, the aim of this workshop is to allow midwives, obstetricians and students to gain experience in the preparation, guidance and communication required to support a woman and her partner during a case of assisted vaginal breech birth. Emphasis is placed on conducting a 'hands off' approach to the birth, but training also covers the specific manoeuvres required to assist with the birth of the baby's legs, arms and head. It also helps staff to be familiar with positions for vaginal breech birth, and also with the location of their emergency birth trolley (containing algorithms/posters for guidance on vaginal breech birth), should an unexpected breech birth occur in the birth centre.

Supporting material

The supporting materials that can be downloaded and printed off are:

- Assisted vaginal breech birth lecture and video
- Vaginal breech birth algorithm
- Maternity notes
- CTG trace and pro forma

Assisted vaginal breech birth scenario

This case presents a 35-year-old woman in her third pregnancy who arrives on the labour ward in spontaneous labour at 37^{+2} weeks of gestation. She has strong urges to push on arrival and the baby is confirmed to be in a breech presentation, with the fetal buttocks presenting just below the ischial spines of the woman's pelvis. The woman is keen to aim for a vaginal birth, so the participants are asked to assist the vaginal birth.

'This is Melissa. She is 35 years old and 37^{+2} weeks pregnant. She has had two vaginal births previously of 3.7 kg and 3.9 kg.

This baby was confirmed on ultrasound yesterday to be in a breech presentation. Melissa was due to come in for an external cephalic version later today but she started contracting 2 hours ago. She has just arrived here on the labour ward and is having strong contractions and urges to push.

I've performed a vaginal examination: the cervix is fully dilated and the buttocks are clearly palpable below the ischial spines. The CTG has been on for 5 minutes so far and there are variable decelerations present. I've discussed these findings with Melissa and she is keen to aim for a vaginal birth.

Melissa is having very strong urges to push now and I can see the fetal buttocks at the introitus. Please could you continue with the birth.'

Equipment

- Patient-actor to integrate with obstetric mannequin
- Maternal and fetal obstetric mannequin, such as the PROMPT Flex (Limbs & Things, UK)
- CTG equipment (cardboard-box CTG machine – see Appendix 3)
- Standard birth/operative vaginal birth pack
- Obstetric forceps (Kielland's and/or Wrigley's)
- Baby towels
- In–out urinary catheter
- Maternity notes, CTG trace and pro forma
- Vaginal breech poster/algorithm (Figure 16.1)
- Laminated clinical checklist and pen

Instructions for drill facilitators

This session can be run as a simulated scenario or as a practical training workshop. It can also be incorporated into the twin birth scenario (Section 17) or the cord prolapse scenario (as this is one of the risks associated with a breech presentation – Section 15).

If possible, integrate a patient-actor with an obstetric mannequin (PROMPT Flex) on a labour ward bed to simulate a vaginal breech scenario. It works well if the patient-actor gently pushes the baby through the maternal

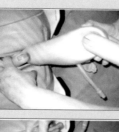
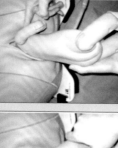
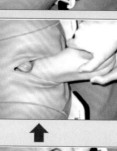
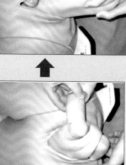
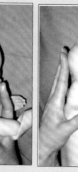
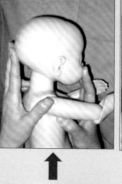
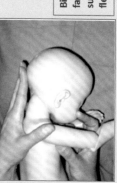
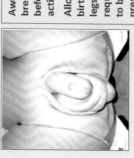

Figure 16.1 Poster demonstrating actions that may be required to assist a vaginal breech birth

mannequin while the accoucheur performs the required manoeuvres. By using a patient-actor, the participant is required to communicate and reassure the mother, thus increasing the realism of the situation.

Simulated scenario

If the scenario is run as a drill, one team member (midwife or junior doctor) should be given the handover information and a printout of the maternity notes, while the rest of the team wait in an appropriate area outside the scenario room until they are called. The faculty members should observe the scenario from a distance, completing the clinical checklist.

Practical workshop

If the scenario is run as a practical hands-on workshop, it should start with a group discussion about the woman's history, followed by a demonstration of a 'hands off' vaginal breech birth as well as the manoeuvres that may be required if assistance is needed. Using the PROMPT vaginal breech birth PowerPoint lecture, and also the pictorial algorithm as part of the session, may help to explain the manoeuvres, and participants should all have hands-on practice during the session.

During the workshop, discuss how the rate of vaginal breech birth has declined over recent years and has continued to decline since the publication of the Term Breech Trial.[1,2,3] However, it remains important for practitioners to maintain their clinical skills to conduct a vaginal breech birth because there will always be situations where a woman presents in advanced labour with a breech presentation (and hence a caesarean section may not be possible), or where a woman may not consent to have an elective caesarean birth. Simulation provides an excellent opportunity to practise these complex but rarely used skills in a safe environment.

Consider the findings of the randomised multicentre Term Breech Trial (2000).[1] Explain that:

- The study compared outcomes after planned vaginal and planned caesarean births for breech presentation and demonstrated a significant reduction in perinatal morbidity and mortality in the planned caesarean group (reduction in mortality of 75%).

- In addition, it was found that there was no significant increase in maternal morbidity or mortality with planned caesarean births.

- However, 2-year follow-up data from the trial did not demonstrate any statistically significant differences in neurodevelopment between the two groups, questioning whether the long-term benefits of planned caesarean birth for breech presentation outweigh the risks.[4]

> ## Recommendations from the RCOG Green-top Guideline for the management of breech presentation (2017)
>
> - When planning a vaginal breech birth, the woman should be informed that the risk of perinatal mortality is approximately 0.5/1000 with caesarean section after 39 weeks of gestation and approximately 2.0/1000 with a planned vaginal breech birth.
>
> - Women should be informed that planned vaginal breech birth increases the risk of low Apgar scores and serious short-term complications, but has not been shown to increase the risk of long-term morbidity.
>
> - Planned caesarean section leads to a small reduction in perinatal mortality compared with planned vaginal breech birth. Any decision to perform a caesarean section needs to be balanced against the potential adverse consequences that may result from this.
>
> - The presence of a skilled birth attendant is essential for a safe vaginal breech birth.
>
> ## Management of preterm singleton breech presentation
>
> - Routine caesarean section for breech presentation in spontaneous preterm labour is not recommended. The mode of birth should be individualised, based on the gestation, stage of labour, type of breech presentation, fetal wellbeing and availability of an operator skilled in vaginal breech birth.
>
> ## Management of twin pregnancy with breech presentation
>
> - Evidence is limited, but if the presenting twin is a breech presentation, then planned caesarean section is recommended.
>
> - Routine emergency caesarean section for a breech presentation of the first twin in spontaneous labour is not recommended. The mode of birth should be individualised, based on cervical dilatation, station of the presenting part, type of breech presentation, fetal wellbeing and availability of an operator skilled in vaginal breech birth.

- This may also be an opportunity to discuss the recent RCOG Green-top Guideline on the management of breech presentation, and how the main emphasis is on the selection of appropriate pregnancies, together with skilled intrapartum care, and how this may allow planned vaginal breech birth to be nearly as safe as planned vaginal cephalic birth (see box).[5]

■ In addition, the facilitator should outline the preparation and organisation required for a vaginal breech birth, including the members of staff that should be present and the equipment needed.

■ It is also vital to emphasise the importance of recommending continuous electronic fetal monitoring with a breech labour. This should continue until birth, even if the decision is taken to perform a caesarean section at any point during labour.

Assisted manoeuvres

HANDS OFF the breech! When demonstrating the assisted manoeuvres required for vaginal breech birth, it is important to emphasise that limited operator handling is crucial, and that as far as possible the baby should be born spontaneously with uterine contractions and maternal effort. However, if handling is necessary, explain that the baby should only be held over the bony prominences of the pelvis to minimise the risk of soft-tissue damage.

Call for help

A senior midwife, obstetrician (experienced in vaginal breech birth) and neonatologist should be asked to attend the birth, with the anaesthetist and theatre team on standby.

Position of mother

Explain that there are limited data in relation to position and outcome for vaginal breech birth. Some experienced obstetricians and midwives have suggested that upright positioning (e.g. mother kneeling on all fours, sitting on a birthing stool, or standing up) may confer some physiological advantages, as well as offering increased maternal choice regarding positioning. However, alternative positions may not currently be familiar to all practitioners, and therefore it remains the responsibility of accoucheurs and also local maternity units as to what positions are recommended in their local practice guidelines.

The updated RCOG guideline recommends that women should be advised that either a semi-recumbent or a forward-facing squatting or all-fours position may be adopted for birth, but positioning should depend on maternal preference and the experience of the attendant. If, however, a forward-facing all-fours position is adopted, then the woman should be advised that recourse to the semi-recumbent position may become necessary if manoeuvres are required, as the accoucheur may be more confident to perform manoeuvres in a dorsal recumbent position.[5]

Explain about evaluating the need for an episiotomy when the perineum is distending and emphasise that it is only indicated to facilitate the birth.

Birth of fetal body and lower limbs

Spontaneous birth of the limbs and body is preferable (Figure 16.2a), but the legs may need to be released by applying pressure to the popliteal fossae (Figure 16.2b).

- Ensure that the buttocks remain sacroanterior. If the body appears to be rotating to a sacroposterior position, controlled rotation may be required, holding the baby over the bony prominences.
- Avoid handling the umbilical cord, as handling will increase vasospasm.
- Encourage spontaneous birth until the scapulae are visible.
- Pulling on the infant's body can cause a nuchal arm and therefore should be avoided.
- If the arms are not released spontaneously, use Løvsett's manoeuvre, as shown and described in Figure 16.3.

Engagement in the pelvis of the after-coming head

After release of the arms, support the baby until the nape of the neck becomes visible, and use the weight of the baby to encourage flexion (Figure 16.4).

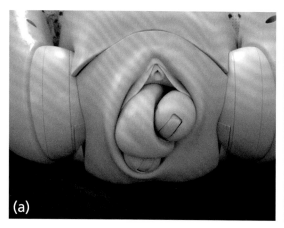
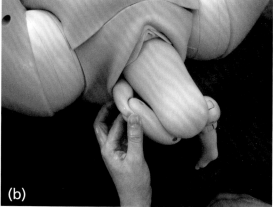

(a)   (b)

Figure 16.2 Release of fetal legs

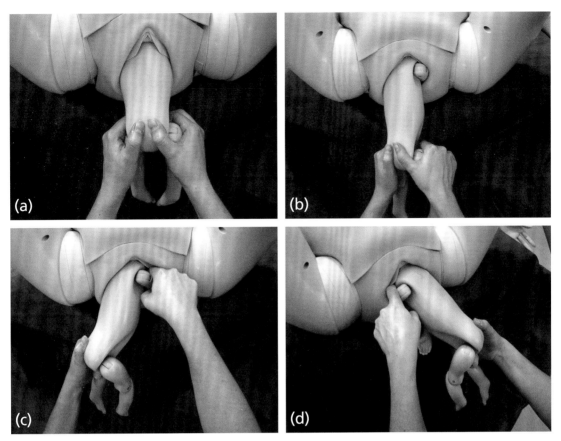

Figure 16.3 Løvsett's manoeuvre. (a) Gently hold the baby over the bony prominences of the hips and sacrum and rotate the baby so that (b) one arm is uppermost (anterior). (c) To release the uppermost arm, an index figure should be placed over the baby's shoulder and follow the arm to the antecubital fossa. The arm should be flexed for delivery. (d) Following release of the first arm, rotate the baby 180 degrees, keeping the back uppermost, so that the second arm is now uppermost. Release this arm as described in (c).

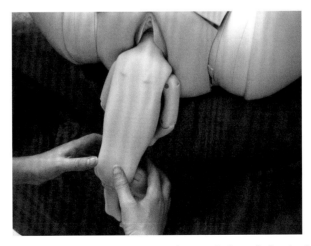

Figure 16.4 Nape of neck visible: using the weight of the baby to encourage flexion

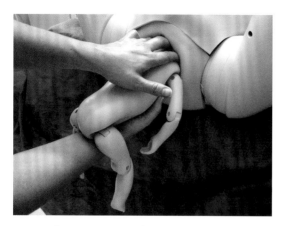

Figure 16.5 The Mauriceau–Smellie–Veit manoeuvre for birth of the after-coming head

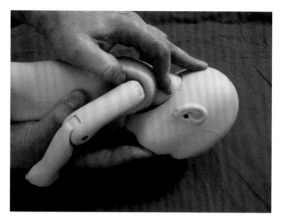

Figure 16.6 Flexion and delivery of the fetal head using the Mauriceau-Smellie-Veit manoeuvre

Mauriceau–Smellie–Veit manoeuvre

The Mauriceau–Smellie–Veit manoeuvre may be required to assist birth of the after-coming head (Figure 16.5). When using this manoeuvre, the baby's body should be supported on the flexor surface of the accoucheur's forearm. The first and third finger of the accoucheur's hand should be placed on the cheekbones (note that the middle finger is no longer placed in the fetal mouth, as fetal injury has been reported). With the other hand, apply pressure to the occiput with the middle finger and place the other fingers simultaneously on the fetal shoulders to promote flexion, i.e. keep the chin on the chest (Figure 16.6).

Also demonstrate that if birth of the head does not follow, an assistant may apply suprapubic pressure to assist flexion of the head (Figure 16.7).[5]

Burns–Marshall technique

There have been some concerns expressed about the risks of the Burns–Marshall method for assisting birth of the head, as it may lead to overextension of the baby's neck. Therefore, it is not advised.

Forceps delivery of the head

Alternatively, the fetal head can be delivered with the aid of forceps. An assistant should hold the baby and the forceps should be applied from underneath the fetal body. The axis of traction should aim to flex the head (Figure 16.8). There is debate over which type of forceps should be used for this procedure, and Kielland's, Rhodes' and Wrigley's forceps have all been reported. It may be useful, if there is time, for the scenario to include the obstetrician applying forceps to the after-coming head, so that all the

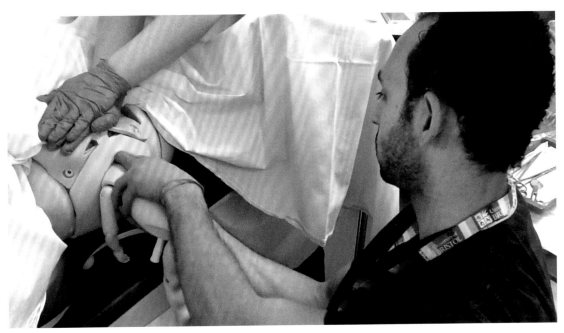

Figure 16.7 Suprapubic pressure applied to assist flexion of the fetal head

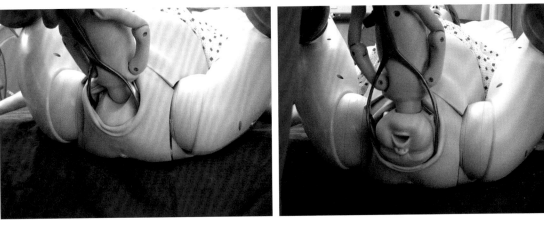

Figure 16.8 Kielland's forceps delivery of the head

maternity staff are familiar with the equipment required, the positioning of the woman (lithotomy position) and support of the attending team.

There is no experimental evidence to indicate which of the above techniques for assisting birth of the fetal head is preferable, and the previous experience of the practitioner will be an important factor in the decision as to which method is chosen.

Complications and potential solutions

Failure to assist birth of the after-coming head

If conservative methods and forceps fail to assist birth of the head, symphysiotomy or caesarean section should be performed. There have been successful births described by both symphysiotomy and rapid caesarean section when attempts to assist birth of the after-coming head have failed.[5]

Head entrapment during a preterm breech birth

The major cause of head entrapment is the passage of the preterm fetal trunk through an incompletely dilated cervix. In this situation, the cervix can be incised to release the head. The incisions should be made at 10 o'clock and 2 o'clock, to avoid the cervical neurovascular bundles that run laterally in the cervix. Care should be taken, as extension into the lower segment of the uterus can occur.

Nuchal arms

Nuchal arm is when one or both of the arms is extended and trapped behind the fetal head, complicating up to 5% of breech births (Figure 16.9). It can be caused by early traction on a breech, which should be avoided as there is a high morbidity associated with nuchal arms, with a 25% risk of neonatal trauma, e.g. brachial plexus injuries.

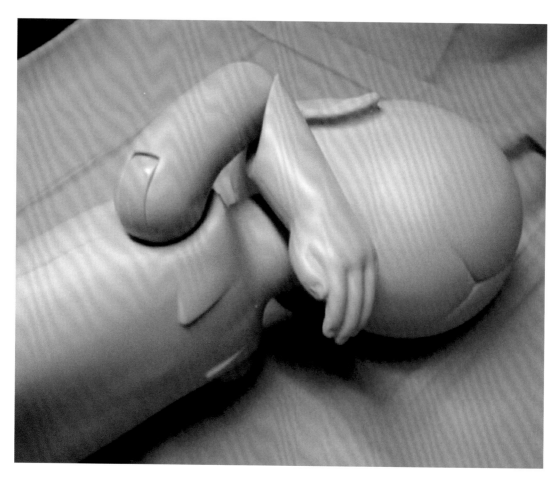

Figure 16.9 Nuchal arm

Nuchal arms can be released using Løvsett's manoeuvre. The accoucheur can run a finger along the arm to the antecubital fossa, applying pressure and flexing the arm to help release it.

Debrief and feedback

Following the scenario, give feedback to the team using the clinical checklist and discuss how the manoeuvres were documented. Teamwork checklists are downloadable and may be used to aid the debrief if the scenario is run as a team drill instead of a workshop. Also ask the patient-actor to comment on how they thought the team acted in terms of:

Respect:	I felt I was treated with respect
Safety:	I felt safe at all times
Communication:	I felt well informed due to good communication

Documentation

The importance of comprehensive and accurate documentation should be emphasised, including persons present at the birth and timings of manoeuvres.

References

1. Hannah ME, Hannah WJ, Hewson SA, *et al.*; Term Breech Trial Collaborative Group. Planned caesarean section versus planned vaginal birth for breech presentation at term: a randomised multicentre trial. *Lancet* 2000; 356: 1375–83.

2. Confidential Enquiry into Stillbirths and Deaths in Infancy. *5th Annual Report*. London: Maternal and Child Health Research Consortium, 1998.

3. Health and Social Care Information Centre. *Hospital Episode Statistics: NHS Maternity Statistics – England 2014–15*. London: HSCIC, 2015. http://content.digital.nhs.uk/catalogue/PUB19127 (accessed August 2017).

4.. Hofmeyr GJ, Hannah M, Lawrie TA. Planned caesarean section for term breech delivery. *Cochrane Database Syst Rev* 2015; (7): CD000166.

5. Royal College of Obstetricians and Gynaecologists. *The Management of Breech Presentation*, 4th edn. Green-top Guideline No. 20B. London: RCOG, 2017. www.rcog.org.uk/en/guide-lines-research-services/guidelines/gtg20B (accessed August 2017).

Assisted vaginal breech birth: clinical checklist

		Time	✔
Call for help	Activate emergency bell Request experienced midwife, experienced obstetrician and neonatologist		
	Request anaesthetist and theatre team to be on standby		
Position of mother	Place mother in semi-recumbent position, or consider forward-facing squatting/all-fours position if birth attendant skilled and trained		
Evaluate for episiotomy	Evaluate for episiotomy when perineum distended by baby's buttocks		
Birth of fetal body and lower limbs	Allow spontaneous birth of the buttocks (hands off)		
	Correct buttocks to sacroanterior		
	Allow spontaneous birth of legs (hands off) but, if not progressing, assist release of legs by applying pressure to popliteal fossae		
	Allow spontaneous birth of body (hands off) until lower scapulae visible		
Birth of arms	Allow spontaneous birth of arms (hands off)		
	If arms require assistance: Gently hold baby over bony prominences of pelvic bones (not abdomen)		
	Keep sacrum/spine anterior		
	Rotate trunk (Løvsett's manoeuvre) and sweep fetal arms down using one or two fingers		
Birth of head	Allow baby to hang so that shoulders and neck descend over next contraction until nape of neck visible (encourages flexion of head)		
	Assist birth of head using Mauriceau–Smellie–Veit or forceps placed on to head from *underneath* body		
Documentation	Persons present		
	Manoeuvres used		
	Timings of actions		

Section 17
Twin birth

Key learning points

- Preparation of room and equipment for twin birth.
- Intrapartum electronic fetal monitoring of both twins.
- Importance of stabilisation of the fetal lie of the second twin.
- To understand the various manoeuvres needed to facilitate birth of the second twin.
- Aim to keep twin-to-twin birth interval to less than 30 minutes.
- Justify situations in which caesarean section may be necessary.
- Recognise the increased risks of postpartum haemorrhage.
- Document details of births accurately, clearly and legibly.

Common difficulties observed in training sessions

- Not setting the room up with the necessary equipment prior to births
- Failure to adequately stabilise and maintain the longitudinal fetal lie of the second twin until the presenting part has engaged into the pelvis
- Premature amniotomy for the second twin

Aims of the twin birth scenario

This workshop is best run as part of a practical training session. It provides an opportunity for the maternity team (midwives, doctors and healthcare assistants) to work through the preparation, guidance and communication required to support a woman and her partner during a vaginal twin birth.

It is important to emphasise the practical nature of the preparation of equipment, using the checklist to help.

Furthermore, there are important clinical aspects of the care that should be highlighted, including the clinical importance of stabilising the lie of the second twin following the birth of the first twin and a justification of a twin-to-twin birth interval of less than 30 minutes. The teaching also covers the specific manoeuvres required to assist with the birth of the second twin and provides an opportunity for hands-on practice using an obstetric mannequin.

Supporting material

The downloadable supporting materials included are:

- Twin birth admission in labour checklist
- Maternity notes
- Twin birth documentation pro forma
- Twin CTG

These are all in a printable format for use in the scenario.

Twin birth scenario

A 29-year-old primiparous woman has been induced at 37 weeks' gestation for a dichorionic, diamniotic twin pregnancy. There has been normal growth and liquor volumes for both twins in her pregnancy. A scan was performed prior to induction that demonstrated that the first twin was a cephalic presentation and the second twin was breech. Both twins have had normal CTGs during labour and the mother has an epidural in place. She is now in the second stage of labour and pushing well; the vertex of the first twin is just visible. The participants are asked to check the equipment required for, and to assist with, the birth of the twins.

> 'Jane is at 37 weeks of gestation and is being induced for a dichorionic, diamniotic twin pregnancy. There has been normal growth and liquor volumes of both twins during pregnancy. A scan was performed prior to induction. Twin I is cephalic and Twin II is breech. She has progressed well in labour, with normal CTGs for both twins. Jane has an epidural in situ and one intravenous line in her arm. She is now fully dilated and is pushing well. The vertex of Twin I is just visible.
>
> Please could you check the equipment and continue with the birth of the twins.'

Equipment

- Patient-actor integrated with obstetric mannequin
- Maternal and fetal obstetric mannequins (with one or two babies), such as the PROMPT Flex Birthing Trainer (Limbs & Things, UK)
- Twin CTG monitor (cardboard-box CTG machine with two fetal heart transducers)
- Standard birth/operative vaginal birth pack
- Forceps and vacuum extraction equipment
- Simulated Syntocinon infusion prepared for augmentation between twin births
- Ultrasound scanner (or laminated photo)
- In–out urinary catheter
- Simulated vial of Syntocinon/Syntometrine for routine active management of the third stage of labour
- Syntocinon vials (normal saline vials re-labelled) and 500 mL normal saline ready for Syntocinon infusion after birth of both twins (for postpartum haemorrhage prophylaxis)
- Blunt needles and syringes
- Amnihook
- Neonatal resuscitation equipment, including baby hats and towels
- Laminated twin birth admission in labour checklist
- Laminated equipment and staff for twin birth checklist
- Laminated twins documentation pro forma and pen
- Laminated clinical checklist and pen

Instructions for drill facilitators

This scenario is best run as part of a hands-on training session. The scenario may also be incorporated with the cord prolapse drill (increased risk in a twin birth) or the vaginal breech birth scenario (second twin is breech in this scenario).

If possible, integrate a patient-actor with an obstetric mannequin on a labour ward bed to simulate a twin birth. It works well if the patient-actor gently pushes each baby through the maternal mannequin while the accoucheur performs the required manoeuvres to assist birth. It is possible to place two babies in the maternal mannequin if they are available; if only one mannequin is available, once the first twin is born it can be passed back to the patient-actor and placed in the maternal mannequin as the second twin in the appropriate position (cephalic, breech or transverse, depending on how you wish the scenario to be managed).

The participants are required to communicate with, and reassure, the mother (patient-actor), which is an essential part of the clinical care.

When the scenario is run as a drill, one team member (midwife or junior doctor) should be given the handover information and printout of the mother's notes, while the rest of the team waits in an appropriate area outside the scenario room until they are called.

Faculty members may observe the scenarios from a distance, completing the clinical checklist.

Practical training session

The practical training session should start with a group discussion about the woman's twin pregnancy and her admission for induction at 37 weeks.

Care in labour

Using the twin birth admission in labour checklist (Figure 17.1), discuss the care and equipment required during labour.

Preparation for twin birth

Emphasise the importance of pre-emptive preparation of the room, including collecting all the equipment required (see box). An ultrasound machine should be ready for use (staff should be aware of where it is usually stored), particularly to check the presentation of Twin II. A laminated photo of the scanner can be used for the training session if the real scanner is in use.

Operative vaginal birth equipment as well as facilities for neonatal resuscitation should be checked and available in the room.

Twin birth: Checklist on admission to labour ward		231
Attach inpatient ID label:	Tick when completed	Comments
Introduce the parents to the team.		
Review the handheld and hospital notes including the care plan to identify any antenatal risk factors.		
Explain the plan for birth.		
Establish intravenous access, take blood for full blood count (FBC) and group and save (G&S).		
Once in established labour for clear fluids only and start gastric protection (e.g. oral Ranitidine 150 mg six-hourly).		
Confirm presentation of both twins with ultrasound.		
Continuous electronic fetal monitoring is recommended: • A scalp electrode may be used for twin I to help differentiate the fetal heart recordings. • Ultrasound can be used to identify the optimal placement of the EFM transducers. • A suitable monitor should be used to enable the differentiation of the two fetal heart tracings.		
Discuss analgesia. An epidural is helpful as it will make any intrauterine manipulation of twin II easier and can be used for caesarean section if needed.		
Obstetrician to document a care plan for twin birth in the handheld record.		
Date: Name: Signature: Grade:		

Figure 17.1 Twin birth: admission in labour checklist

Discuss the need for experienced staff to be present at the birth of twins. These should include: two midwives, an obstetrician, neonatal staff (particularly for Twin II), and an anaesthetist and theatre team present on the labour ward.

Equipment required for a twin birth

- Ultrasound scanner
- Lithotomy supports
- Amnihook
- Local anaesthetic (e.g. 20 mL 1% lidocaine), syringe and needle
- Operative vaginal birth trolley
- Forceps and ventouse
- Birth instruments pack
- Additional set of cord clamps
- Four cord blood sampling syringes
- Two resuscitaires (labelled Twin I and Twin II)
- Two sets of warmed baby towels and hats
- Oxytocin infusion for augmentation (e.g. 3 units Syntocinon in 50 mL normal saline) ready to be commenced after the birth of the first twin, if required
- Syntocinon or Syntometrine for third stage of labour as appropriate
- Oxytocin infusion (e.g. 40 units Syntocinon in 500 mL normal saline) for prophylactic use after the third stage, but kept separately from the oxytocin infusion used between the first and second twin

Birth of the second twin

Explain that once the first twin has been born (assisted by the midwife, if a normal birth), it is important to have an experienced member of staff allocated to the task of stabilising the lie of the second twin in a longitudinal lie. A Syntocinon infusion should be prepared and ready to augment the contractions in case there is a reduction in their frequency between the two births. Also, explain the importance of waiting until the presenting part of the second twin has descended into the pelvis before rupturing the membranes, to avoid a preventable cord prolapse. Emphasise that ideally the second twin should be born within 30 minutes of the first twin, and that birth should be expedited if the birth of the second twin is delayed and/or there is fetal compromise.

Finally, discuss the management of a second twin in a transverse or oblique lie. There are two options described in the *Course Manual*:

- External cephalic version
- Internal podalic version

External cephalic version

When attempting external cephalic version (Figure 17.2), demonstrate how the ultrasound probe can be used as a 'hand' so that fetal lie and heart rate can be monitored throughout.

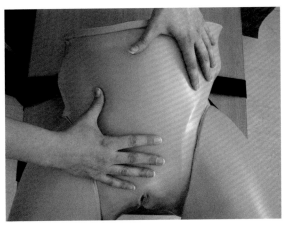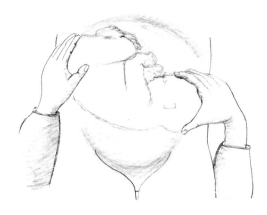

Figure 17.2 External cephalic version

Internal podalic version

One or both fetal feet are grasped inside the uterus and delivered through the cervix, before proceeding to a breech extraction (Figure 17.3). Before any traction is applied, the operator must confirm that he/she is holding a foot by feeling the heel (90-degree angle, which a hand does not have). Once again, it is important to avoid hasty or premature rupture of the membranes until the presenting part of the second twin is in the pelvis, to avoid a preventable cord prolapse.

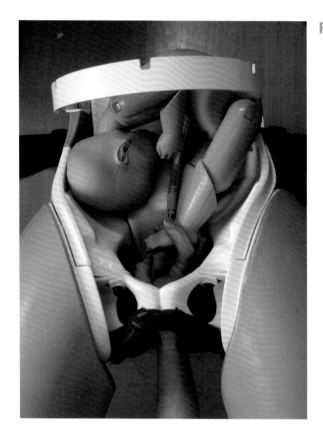

Figure 17.3 Internal podalic version

Assisted vaginal breech birth

The manoeuvres described in **Section 16** (*Vaginal breech birth*) can be demonstrated for the assisted vaginal breech birth of Twin II.

Active management of third stage

Finally, discuss that there is currently insufficient evidence to make any recommendation about delayed cord clamping with twin births. However, there is a high risk of postpartum haemorrhage owing to a large uterus and large placental site. Therefore, it is important to recommend active management of the third stage and commence a prophylactic Syntocinon infusion after completion of the third stage, to reduce the risk of PPH.

Documentation

The importance of comprehensive and accurate documentation should be emphasised, including noting all of the maternity team present, and the times and modes of both births. Figure 17.4 provides an example of a twin birth documentation pro forma.

Twin birth – Documentation pro forma			
Name:	**Hospital Number:**		**Date:**
Gestation:			Comments:
Chorionicity	Dichorionic/diamniotic or Monochorionic/diamniotic		
	Twin I	**Twin II**	
Presentation at start of 2nd stage	Cephalic Breech Other	Cephalic Breech Other	
CTG	Normal Suspicious Pathological	Normal Suspicious Pathological	
Syntocinon infusion to augment labour?	Yes No	Yes No	
Analgesia	None Entonox Epidural Spinal GA	None Entonox Epidural Spinal GA	
IV access?	Yes No If no, reason for no access:		
Ranitidine?	Yes: oral IV No		
Senior midwife present?	Yes Name: No		
Obstetric registrar (ST3–5) present?	Yes Name: No		
Senior obstetric registrar (ST6–7)?	Yes Name: No		
Consultant obstetrician present?	Yes Name: No		
Experienced neonatologist present at birth?	Yes Name: No		
Mode of birth twin I **Time:**	Spontaneous vaginal Ventouse	Forceps Caesarean section	
Syntocinon infusion between twins?	Yes	No	
Mode of birth twin II **Time:**	Spontaneous vaginal Ventouse Forceps	Caesarean section Assisted breech Breech extraction	
	Twin I	**Twin II**	
Presentation at birth	Cephalic Breech Other	Cephalic Breech Other	
Internal or external manoeuvres performed	Yes: No	Yes: No	
Cord gases taken?	Yes No	Yes No	
Apgars (at 1, 5, 10 minutes)			
Placenta complete? (Placenta should be sent to histology)	Yes: No:	Yes: No:	
Syntocinon infusion commenced after third stage?	Yes: No:		
Date: **Name:**	**Signature:**		**Grade:**

Figure 17.4 Example of a twin birth documentation pro forma

Debrief and feedback

Whether this scenario is run as a workshop or as a drill, the twin birth clinical checklist may be used to facilitate discussion and feedback. Teamwork checklists can also be used to facilitate the debrief when the scenario is run as a team drill, instead of a preparation and management workshop.

Twin birth: clinical checklist

		Time	✓
Equipment preparation	2 × resuscitaires Ultrasound scanner Operative vaginal birth trolley Amnihook Venflon with sharps removed Syntocinon infusion for augmentation between birth of Twin I and Twin II Syntocinon infusion for PPH prophylaxis		
Persons present	2 × midwives Experienced obstetrician 2 × persons trained in neonatal resuscitation Obstetric anaesthetist and theatre staff present on labour ward		
Stabilising lie of second twin	Using ultrasound		
Commencing syntocinon infusion between twin births	Ensuring IV access Syntocinon infusion ready in infusion pump		
Rupturing membranes	Not performing ARM too early		
External cephalic version or internal podalic version (if necessary)	Understand manoeuvres required		
Assisted breech birth (if necessary)	Use PROMPT vaginal breech birth clinical checklist		
Active management of third stage	IM Syntometrine Syntocinon infusion for PPH prophylaxis according to local protocol		
Documentation	Timings of actions		
	Use of documentation pro forma		

Section 18

Acute uterine inversion

Common difficulties observed in training drills

- Delay in recognition of uterine inversion
- Not stating the problem clearly to those first attending the emergency call
- Delay in commencing resuscitation
- Delay in manually replacing the uterus
- Not being prepared for a subsequent postpartum haemorrhage

Aims of the uterine inversion scenario

The aim of this scenario is to allow the multi-professional obstetric team to gain experience of the immediate management of an acute uterine inversion. This is a rare obstetric emergency, and delayed recognition of the problem can lead to complications. The emphasis of this scenario is therefore on recognising the clinical signs and symptoms associated with uterine inversion, as well as the immediate management required to replace the uterus and resuscitate the woman.

It is also important that the participants recognise the inevitable problem of postpartum haemorrhage (PPH) associated with uterine inversion, and the need to make safe plans for manual removal of the placenta after the uterus has been replaced.

Supporting material

The downloadable supporting materials included are:

- Treatment algorithms for the management of acute uterine inversion and PPH
- Maternity notes

These are all in a printable format for use in the scenario.

Acute uterine inversion scenario

This case presents a 30-year-old multiparous woman who gave birth to her third baby half an hour ago. There has already been an unsuccessful attempt at delivering the placenta and the midwife is asked to continue. As controlled cord traction is attempted, the uterus will invert.

After the handover, the woman should say that she is in pain, and that she feels something might be pushing down. The team member taking over should then start to perform controlled cord traction by pulling on the simulated cord. This will result in a uterine inversion, causing the patient-actor to shout in pain, feel very unwell and then collapse.

The team member should call for help and, once the uterine inversion is recognised, the placenta and uterus should be easily replaced. However, once replaced, vaginal bleeding will develop and PPH will ensue unless effective preventive treatment is established.

This module can be used in conjunction with the PPH algorithms and checklists found in **Section 12** (*Major obstetric haemorrhage*).

The drill will end when the woman is stabilised and the decision for transfer to theatre for manual removal of the placenta has been made.

> 'This is Carol, who has just given birth to Alfie, her third baby, about 30 minutes ago. She has had Syntocinon 10 units intramuscularly for the third stage of labour; however, the placenta has not yet delivered, despite attempting controlled cord traction.
>
> Carol has had a blood loss of about 350 mL in total so far and all of her observations have been normal. I think Carol's perineum is intact, but we will need to check fully once the placenta is out.
>
> She had a very rapid labour of only 45 minutes, just arriving in hospital in time to give birth. Alfie weighed 4.0 kg, and he has been skin to skin and is breastfeeding well.
>
> Carol, I have noticed that there seems to be more blood loss now, so we really need to help you to get this placenta out. Is that OK with you?'

Equipment

- SimMom full-body mannequin (Laerdal Medical, Norway) set up for inverted uterus scenario (see user's manual); or
- Patient-actor sat upright in labour ward bed holding the baby doll wrapped in blanket, wearing the 'magic trousers' as used in the PPH scenario, and with a 'magic cushion' (a cushion with a fabric uterus that inverts) inserted inside the trousers (see **Appendix 3** for details of these props)
- Sphygmomanometer/automated blood pressure machine
- IV cannulae with sharps removed
- Blood bottles and forms
- Oxygen mask with reservoir bag and tubing
- IV fluids and giving sets
- Infusion pumps or laminated pictures
- Simulated drugs (could be 0.9% saline ampoules re-labelled):
  - ☐ terbutaline/GTN (for replacement of the uterus)

☐ oxytocin/ergometrine/Syntometrine/carboprost (for prevention/ treatment of PPH)

■ Maternity notes

■ MOEWS chart

■ Local medication and fluid charts, and consent form

■ Clock for documentation of timings

■ Laminated management of uterine inversion algorithm

■ Laminated management of PPH algorithm

■ Laminated clinical and teamwork checklists and pens

Instructions for drill facilitators

The handover should be given to a member of staff (a midwife or obstetrician) and they should be prompted to perform controlled cord traction to complete the third stage of labour (the rest of the team should be waiting in an appropriate area outside the room).

If there is a team observing, they should be given clinical and teamwork checklists to complete and asked to stand in the corner of the labour room. If there is no observing team, the faculty should complete the checklists.

When the team member attempts controlled cord traction, the simulated uterus will invert through the magic trousers with the placenta remaining attached, and the patient-actor will collapse (Figure 18.1). The team member can easily replace the uterus by pushing it back into the cushion to which it is attached.

	Baseline	On inverting the uterus	PPH with uterus replaced	PPH with uterus inverted
Heart rate (bpm)	80	49	105	90
Blood pressure (mmHg)	120/60	80/50	95/60	70/40
Respiratory rate	18			
SpO$_2$	100			
Temperature (°C)	37			

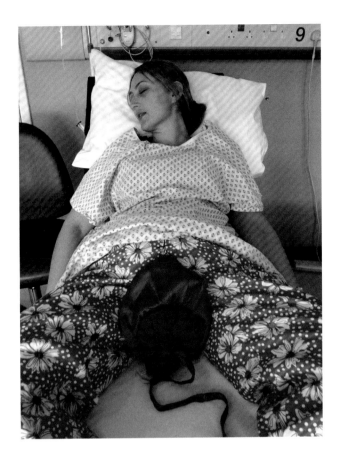

Figure 18.1 Patient-actor collapsed after simulated uterine inversion (wearing magic trousers)

After replacement of the uterus, or after 1 or 2 minutes if the team does not recognise the inverted uterus, the red cloth from the magic trousers should be intermittently pulled out to simulate haemorrhage.

If the observations are checked during the scenario, the team should be informed of the readings as outlined in the table. If the uterus has been replaced, and there is appropriate fluid resuscitation, then the observations should improve, even with a PPH; however, hypotension should persist despite fluid therapy if the uterus has not been replaced (neurogenic shock).

The team is expected to recognise the uterine inversion, call for help and initiate basic actions. This should include placing the baby safely in a cot, lying the woman flat, administering oxygen, immediately replacing the uterus, and commencing fluid resuscitation as outlined in the uterine inversion algorithm (Figure 18.2). The team should start medication to prevent or treat PPH and should consider transfer to theatre for manual

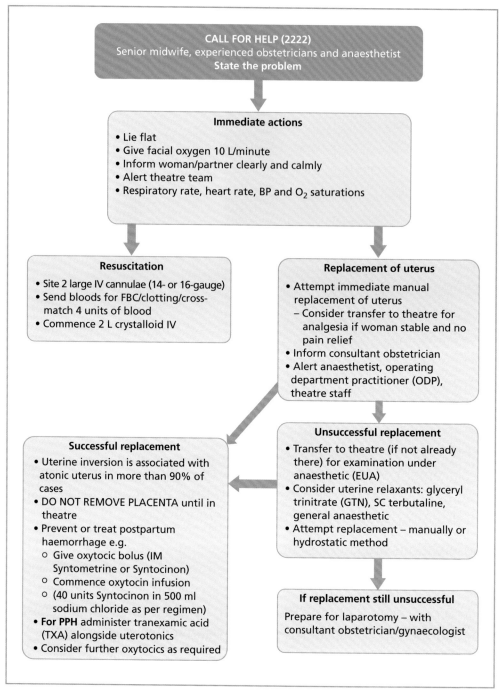

Figure 18.2 Algorithm for the management of uterine inversion

removal of the placenta. If team members are unsure about performing the necessary actions, the prompts outlined below may be used to guide the scenario.

The drill will end when the woman is stabilised and the decision for transfer to theatre has been made.

Prompts

If no attempt to deliver the placenta:	'Do you think you can deliver the placenta now?'
If inverted uterus is not recognised:	'What do you think the problem is?' Red cloth should be pulled out of trousers to simulate bleeding after 1–2 minutes
If the team call for help:	'Who do you need?'
If resuscitation is not commenced:	'Is there anything you can do to help Carol?'
If blood is taken and results requested:	'The results are not yet available.'
If request to transfer to theatre before uterine replacement/stabilisation/treatment for haemorrhage commenced:	'Theatres are busy for at least the next 20 minutes. Is there anything else you can do here?'

Instructions for the patient-actor

When the team member attempts to deliver the placenta, the simulated uterus will invert from the magic cushion and through the magic trousers. As this happens you should pretend to feel unwell, start to faint and release your grip on the baby.

The team may try to replace the uterus by pushing it back inside the cushion to which it is attached; as this is performed you should moan as if in pain.

After replacement of the uterus, or after 1–2 minutes, if the team does not recognise inversion of the uterus, you should intermittently pull out lengths of the red cloth from the leg of the magic trousers to simulate haemorrhage.

Debrief and feedback

After the drill, clinical and teamwork checklists should be reviewed to guide the debrief of team actions. Group discussion should also cover:

- Signs and symptoms of uterine inversion, including recognising neurogenic shock
- Methods of replacing the inverted uterus, including medications and the hydrostatic technique (refer to Module 14 in the *Course Manual*)
- Risk of PPH and treatments required

The patient-actor should also be asked for feedback about how they thought the team acted in terms of:

Respect:	I felt I was treated with respect
Safety:	I felt safe at all times
Communication:	I felt well informed due to good communication

Uterine inversion scenario: clinical checklist

		Time	✓
Call for help	Emergency call bell – request experienced help		
	State the problem		
Airway	Maintain airway		
Breathing	Check breathing		
	Administer full-flow oxygen		
Circulation	Lie flat or head down		
	Insert 2 large-gauge cannulae		
	Take bloods for FBC, clotting and cross-match 4 units		
Fluids	Commence IV fluids		
Treatment	**Treatment for uterine inversion** Inform consultant obstetrician Immediate manual replacement of uterus if possible. 　▪ Consider transfer to theatre for anaesthetic 　▪ Consider tocolytic 　▪ Consider hydrostatic replacement Transfer to theatre for manual removal of placenta		
	Treatment for haemorrhage Uterine massage/bimanual compression Oxytocic bolus, e.g. Syntometrine/Syntocinon Oxytocin infusion Tranexamic acid (alongside uterotonics) Intramuscular carboprost Misoprostol per rectum (if refrigerated tocolytics unavailable) Empty bladder Keep woman warm		
Monitoring	Measure pulse, respiration, O_2 saturations and blood pressure		
	Use MOEWS chart or maternal critical care chart (adapted MOEWS)		
	Urinary catheter and hourly measurements		
Inspection	Measure blood loss		
	Uterine tone		
	Placenta and membranes		
Documentation	Timings of events		
	Observations and fluid balance		
	Medication administered		
	Persons present		

Uterine inversion scenario: teamwork checklists

Communication		YES	NO
State the problem	Clinical problem was stated clearly to arriving team		
Instructions	Instructions were clearly worded		
	Unnecessary conversation/noise was avoided		
	Action plans were shared		
	Goals were clearly identified		
Addressed	Specific instructions were given to the appropriate team members		
Sent	Communication was not rushed		
	It was clear what action was required		
Heard	Acknowledgements were made		
	Requests for repeat information were made		
Understood	The information was understood and repeated back by recipient		
	The correct action was performed		

Team roles and leadership		YES	NO
Roles	Each team member had a clear role		
	There was a team leader		
Adaptability	Team members responded well to different situations		
Responsibility	Team members assumed responsibility for their role		
Advocate	Tasks were delegated appropriately		
Feedback	There were regular updates on progress		
	A running commentary was provided		
Support	Team members did not argue about issues		
	None of the team members decided to 'go it alone'		

Situational awareness/standing back, taking a broader view		YES	NO
Notice	There was an awareness of what each member of the team was doing		
	There was an awareness of the resources that were needed		
	Mistakes were identified		
Understand	Regular updates took place throughout the scenario		
	Problems were identified		
	A re-evaluation was undertaken		
	Team members were asked for their opinion		
	Team members were asked to suggest possible solutions		
	A clear action plan was made		
Prioritise	Key tasks were given priority		
Delegate	Each team member had a specific task		
	The tasks were delegated appropriately		

Section 19

Basic newborn resuscitation and support of transition

Key learning points

- To develop and rehearse a structured approach to the individual and team skills required in neonatal resuscitation.
- To understand that the primary aim of newborn resuscitation is inflation of the lungs with air or oxygen: inflation breaths followed by additional ventilations (ensuring good chest movement) should, in itself, increase the infant's heart rate.
- To understand the importance of calling for help early.
- To understand the importance of keeping the baby warm.
- To communicate effectively with all members of the maternity and neonatal team.
- To include communication with the parents during the emergency and ensure debriefing afterwards.

Common difficulties observed in training drills

- Poor thermal care during resuscitation, especially in preterm infants
- Failure to open the infant's airway adequately, usually due to over-extension of the neck
- Failing to maintain an effective airway, particularly when conducting simultaneous cardiac compressions

- Performing chest compressions too slowly
- Poor communication and leadership within the multi-professional team

Aims of the newborn resuscitation scenarios

There are three scenarios included, each with a different clinical issue around the mode or place of birth of the infant. The scenarios will enable midwives, obstetricians, neonatologists, advanced neonatal nurse practitioners and healthcare support workers, as well as student midwives and doctors, to learn the practical skills and experience required for effective basic newborn resuscitation in a simulated birth setting. The scenarios are intended for local training use, and should act as an adjunct to formal newborn life support courses.

Supporting material

The downloadable supporting materials included are:

- Basic newborn resuscitation algorithm
- Clinical checklist

Scenarios

The three cases represent a newborn infant requiring:

1. Initial resuscitation following an operative vaginal birth
2. Initial resuscitation where there is meconium
3. Resuscitation in a home setting, until help arrives

Equipment

- Resuscitaire or home birth neonatal resuscitation equipment
- Resuscitation mannequin, e.g. Resusci Baby or NeoNatalie (Laerdal, Norway)
- 3 × towels/blankets and baby hats

- Neonatal bag-valve-mask
- 2 × different sizes neonatal face mask
- 3 × different sizes neonatal Guedel airways (2.5, 3.0, 3.5)
- Suction tubing and suction catheter for neontatal use
- Neonatal Yankaer sucker
- T-piece tubing/Neopuff circuit and connector
- 2 × different sizes neonatal laryngoscope
- Local neonatal notes for documentation

Setting-up instructions

The faculty should include a neonatologist and/or a midwife who has attended the Newborn Life Support Course (Resuscitation Council, UK). Allocate one of the team members to complete the clinical checklist. Use the modified algorithm provided for newborn life support (Figure 19.1) to prompt and guide where needed.

Scenario 1

'You are called to attend an operative vaginal birth for prolonged fetal bradycardia of a term infant. The neonatologist has been called but has not yet arrived. The resuscitaire has been checked and prepared with the heater on and towels warming. A baby boy has just been born using mid-cavity forceps. He is floppy and white, his heart rate is slow and he is making no respiratory effort.'

Actions

1. The participant should:

      - Call urgently for neonatologist
      - Take the infant to the resuscitaire and place him flat on his back
      - Start the clock on the resucitaire
      - Dry and stimulate the infant using a warm towel; discard the wet towel and wrap in another dry towel
      - Assess the infant's colour, heart rate, breathing and tone

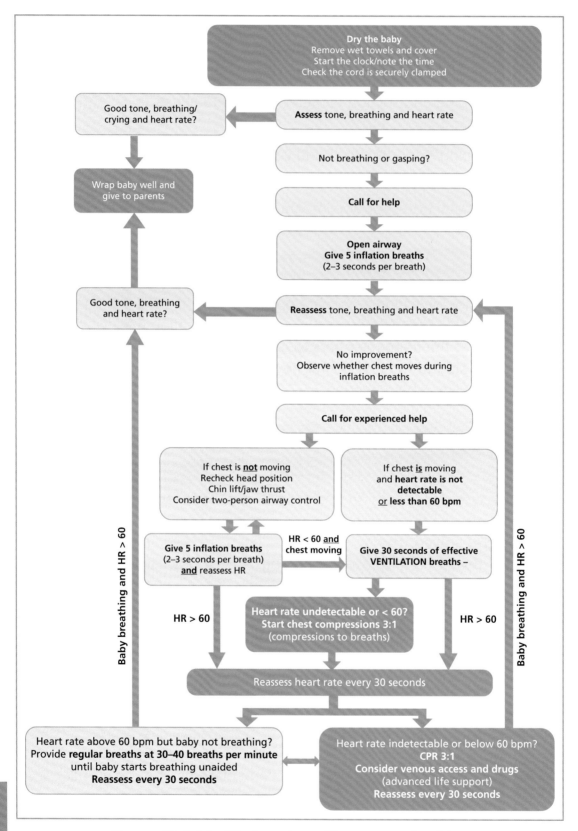

Figure 19.1 Modified newborn life support algorithm

■ Maintain infant's head in a *neutral* position to establish a clear airway

■ Give five inflation breaths

2. If the heart rate remains slow:

■ The participant should request urgent senior neonatal support if not already in attendance.

■ If the inflation breaths are not effective at inflating the chest (a common problem), the participant should adjust the position of the infant's head and give a further five inflation breaths.

■ If the inflation breaths were effective at inflating the chest (the participant should state that chest movement was seen), the participant should now administer 30 seconds of ventilation breaths, then reassess.

■ If the heart rate still remains slow, commence chest compressions: three compressions to one breath (3:1).

3. If chest compressions are effective after two cycles and the baby's heart rate begins to rise, the facilitator should explain that both the infant's colour and tone are improving and he is now blue instead of white.

4. Ventilation breaths should be continued, and the facilitator should explain that the infant is now pink but still has minimal respiratory effort.

5. The participant should continue to support ventilation until further senior neonatal support arrives.

Scenario 2

'You have been called to help at a birth where there is thick meconium-stained liquor present. The baby is 37 weeks' gestation. The neonatologist has been called but is unable to attend straight away. At birth, the baby girl appears blue with no initial respiratory effort. The baby's heart rate is slow (less than 100 bpm)'

Actions

1. The participant should immediately prepare and check the resuscitaire, followed by the other equipment, while awaiting the birth.

2. The heater should be switched on and towels should be warming.

3. At birth, the clock on the resuscitaire should be started and the infant should be immediately covered. If thick meconium is present do not

rub or stimulate the baby. Lung inflation within the first minute is the priority and should not be delayed. If the baby is unresponsive and the participant is NLS trained, then they may use a laryngoscope to visualise the vocal cords, and use suction to remove any visible meconium. **Blind suctioning should not be carried out**. If the participant is not trained to use a laryngoscope, only the mouth and nose should be suctioned. The baby should then be dried and stimulated with the warmed towels. Any wet towels should be discarded; the baby should then be wrapped in dry, warmed blankets and a hat placed on her head.

4. The neonatologist should be called again urgently. The infant's colour, heart rate, breathing and tone should be reassessed.

5. If there is still no respiratory effort after rubbing and drying, the participant should check that the infant's head is in the neutral position so that the airway is open, and check the heart rate again.

6. If the heart rate is slow and there is still no respiratory effort, senior neonatal support should be called.

7. The participant should then continue resuscitation, commencing with five inflation breaths, as per the neonatal resuscitation algorithm. If resuscitation is performed appropriately, the heart rate will rise and respiratory effort will start after 30 seconds of ventilation breaths. If resuscitation is performed inadequately or inappropriately, the heart rate may fall and cardiac massage will be required. If this is performed, the situation improves after one cycle of CPR (3 compressions : 1 ventilation – 120 events per minute)

8. The participant should continue ventilation breaths until help arrives.

Scenario 3

This scenario can be carried out as if at a home birth, using basic neonatal resuscitation equipment (bag-valve-mask, neonatal Guedel airway, stopwatch). Two patient-actors could act as the anxious parents of the infant, so that the participants can practise communication with the parents as they manage the resuscitation.

'You are attending a planned home birth. A female infant is born within minutes of arrival after a precipitate labour and birth. The baby girl is given immediately to mum for skin-to-skin contact but she appears to be blue and is gasping.'

Actions

1. The participants (midwife and colleague) should explain that, if there is time, some towels should be placed on the radiator to warm and the home birth emergency neonatal resuscitation equipment should be checked and set up ready near to the birth area.

2. At birth, the time should be noted or a stopwatch could be started (if available).

3. As the baby girl is placed skin-to skin, she should be dried and a warm dry towel placed over her. The midwife should assess the infant's colour, heart rate, breathing and tone.

4. The facilitator should announce that there has been no improvement in the heart rate after 1 minute. The participants should explain to the parents that their baby needs to be given help with her breathing and that they will need to take the baby to the resuscitation area for this to be done.

5. The second participant should call an emergency ambulance, explaining that they have a newborn baby requiring resuscitation and they will need to transfer the mother and baby to hospital. This should also be explained to the parents.

6. The infant should be wrapped up and rubbed vigorously (and hat put on) in the resuscitation area, explaining all actions to the parents. If there is still no respiratory effort after rubbing vigorously, the heart rate should be checked. If the heart rate is rising but there is still little respiratory effort, the infant's head should be maintained in the neutral position and five inflation breaths given. If the inflation breaths are effective, the infant should quickly improve, commence breathing and start to cry normally. If the inflation breaths are ineffective, then a further five breaths should be given after adjusting the infant's head into the neutral position. Following these additional breaths, the baby will begin to breathe regularly.

Debrief and feedback

At the end of each scenario, remind participants that most babies will be born in good condition and will need no more than drying and stimulation at birth.

Remind participants to think ahead about why a baby may be compromised at birth – has there been an APH, are there signs of sepsis, or a pathological CTG? Emphasise the importance of preparing resuscitation equipment in advance and calling for neonatal support early, especially at a home birth or in a standalone birth suite where the nearest neonatologist is an ambulance ride away. In these circumstances, you could also discuss the importance of ringing ahead to inform the labour ward that you are on your way in, so that they can prepare equipment and have appropriate neonatal staff ready for the baby's arrival at the maternity unit.

Using the clinical checklist, ask the observer to feed back. Then talk through the resuscitation steps again, ensuring that those not participating in the drill are given a chance of hands-on experience of resuscitating a neonate.

Stress the importance of always assessing the fetal tone, colour, breathing and heart rate in the first minute after birth, and that if a baby does require resuscitation, the most important thing is to ensure adequate ventilation.

Almost all babies will respond to five effective inflation breaths. The skill is to ensure that the inflation breaths are effective. The participants should all be able to demonstrate that they can maintain an open airway in a neonate and effectively inflate the lungs. Participants must practise opening the airway by placing the baby's head in the neutral position (Figures 19.2 and 19.3), performing a chin lift and jaw thrust (Figure 19.4) and giving effective inflation breaths using the correct-size mask (Figure 19.5).

At this stage, it is also important to discuss the new addition to the Resuscitation Council (UK) guidance of administering 30 seconds of ventilations, if after 5 effective inflation breaths the heart rate has not increased, **before starting chest compressions**.[1]

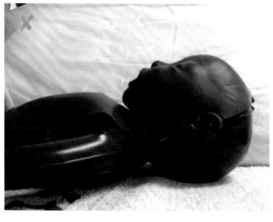

Figure 19.2 Airway obstruction caused by prominent occiput

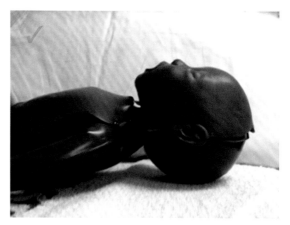

Figure 19.3 Head in the neutral position, opening the airway

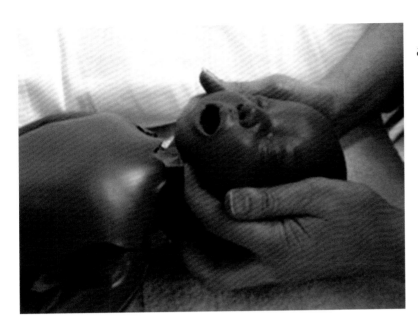

Figure 19.4 Chin lift and jaw thrust to open the airway

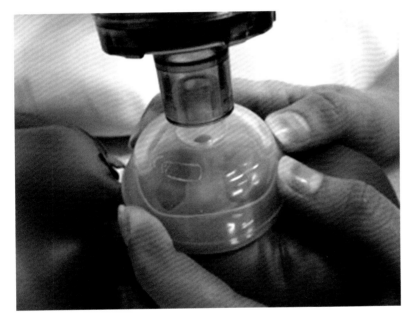

Figure 19.5 Inflation breaths using correct-sized face mask covering the nose and mouth

Remind participants that term babies should no longer be resuscitated with oxygen, and that resuscitation should always be commenced in air.

If chest compressions are required, make sure that the ventilation breaths given are effective, and practise this in the debrief, as participants can often 'lose' the airway when compressions are performed.

Also remind participants that if a baby is compromised at birth, they need to ensure that the umbilical cord is double-clamped so that blood can be taken for cord pH measurements.

Women and Children's Health

NEONATAL RESUSCITATION DOCUMENTATION

North Bristol *NHS*
NHS Trust

Date ....Time ....

Mother

Affix small addressograph
(Name, Hospital Number, DOB)

Person completing form ....

Designation ....Signature ....

Baby

Affix small addressograph
(Name, Hospital Number, DOB)

Called for Help at:

Name of staff present	Role	Time of arrival

APGAR SCORE	1min	5min	10min	15min
Heart rate				
Respiration				
Muscle Tone				
Reflex Response				
Colour				
TOTAL				

Time of birth: ....

Mode of birth: ....

Heart Rate at Birth: ....

Time heart rate above 100 bpm: ....

Time of onset of regular respirations: ....

O2 SATS: ....

Risk factors (GBS, Prom, Mec, Maternal temp) ....

If mother transferred from the birth centre or home please complete the following:

Was an Ambulance required	Time Ambulance called	Time Ambulance arrived birth centre/ home	Time Ambulance left birth centre/home	Time arrived at Hospital

Procedure carried out	Tick	Time	By whom	Comments/ details of the baby's response (comment on changes in HR, colour or resps)
Cord clamped and cut				
Baby dried and stimulated				
5 Inflation Breaths				
Ventilation Breaths				
Cardiac compressions				
Any other procedures				
Intubated? Central Access?				

Emergency drugs (can be given in any order under the direction of a neonatologist)

Drugs are needed rarely and only if there is no significant cardiac output despite effective lung inflation and chest compression.

Adrenaline   **0.1 ml/kg of 1:10,000.** *Can go up to a dose of up to 30 mcg kg-1 (0.3 ml kg-1 of 1:10,000 solution) may be tried.*

Sodium bicarbonate 4.2%   **2-4 ml/kg** *(1-2 mmol/kg 4.2% bicarbonate solution).*

10% Dextrose   **2.5 ml/kg**

0.9% Sodium Chloride   **10 ml/kg of or O negative blood**

Drugs Used	Times given

O Neg blood given?	Y/N
Time	

Blood transfusion lab informed (tick) ☐

eAIMS completed? ....

Cord gases: Art pH.........   Art BE..........   Venous pH..........   Venous BE..........   Lactate...........

Figure 19.6 An example of a neonatal resuscitation documentation pro forma

Timely cord clamping

With regard to timely cord clamping, discuss that there is insufficient evidence to recommend an appropriate time for clamping the cord in babies who are severely compromised at birth. Therefore, for babies requiring resuscitation, resuscitative interventions must remain a priority.

Communication with parents and documentation

If you included patient-actors to play the mother or parents of the infant in the scenario, you may wish to ask them to feed back on the communication and explanations that they received.

Finally, it is important to discuss documentation. The team may have allocated a scribe during the scenario, or they may document timings, people present and actions taken once the infant has been resuscitated. They could even use the clinical checklist/resuscitation pro forma for documenting events (see an example in Figure 19.6). They would of course still need to complete their own local neonatal notes. It is essential to document that 'chest movement was seen' when documenting that five inflation breaths were given.

Further information can be found in the Resuscitation Council (UK) guidelines.[1]

Reference

1.   Resuscitation Council (UK). Resuscitation and support of transition of babies at birth. *Resuscitation Guidelines* 2015. www.resus.org.uk/resuscitation-guidelines/resuscitation-and-support-of-transition-of-babies-at-birth/ (accessed August 2017).

Basic newborn resuscitation scenario: clinical checklist

		Time	✓
Preparation	Awareness of risk factors		
	Preparation of equipment		
	Request neonatologist		
	Warm towels		
	Ensure clock working		
Assessment of baby at birth	Dry and rub the baby		
	Start the clock		
	Remove wet towels and wrap in dry towel and hat		
	Assess colour, tone, breathing and heart rate		
Call for help	Emergency bell activated/paramedic ambulance		
Airway	Position infant on back with head in neutral position		
	Assess if chin lift and/or jaw thrust are required		
	If infant unresponsive and thick meconium present: suction below cords under direct vision using laryngoscope (if trained), or just suction nose and mouth if not trained		
Breathing	Check breathing		
	If not breathing or low heart rate: give five effective inflation breaths		
	Observe for passive chest movement with inflation breaths		
	If no chest movement: adjust head position to open airway and give a further five inflation breaths		
	If heart rate increases but there is no breathing, commence ventilation breaths at 30–40/minute		
Circulation	If heart rate slow or absent after five **effective** breaths, give 30 seconds of ventilation breaths. Reassess, and if heart rate remains slow, commence chest compressions		
	3 compressions : 1 ventilation		
	Aim for 90 compressions and 30 ventilations in every minute (120 events per minute)		
Documentation	Timings of events		
	Actions performed		
	Persons present		

Appendix 1
Example PROMPT course programmes

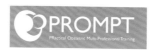

Example PROMPT course programme 1

Time	Programme	Format	Trainer/s
08.30	**Tea/coffee and registration**		
08.45	Introduction to course with team working Includes 'ice breaker'	Lecture	
09.15	Basic life support (all teams)	Instruction	
09.45	Severe hypertension/eclampsia scenario + teamwork	Drill	
10.00	Hypertensive disorders in pregnancy	Lecture	
10.30	Severe hypertension/eclampsia scenario + teamwork (observing and participating teams swap round)	Drill	
10.45	Debrief (all teams)		
11.00	**Tea/coffee break**		
11.15	Maternal critical care and cardiac disorders	Lecture	
11.45	Recognition of the unwell pregnant woman + teamwork	Drill	
12.00	Sepsis, recognition of the unwell pregnant woman	Lecture	
12.30	Recognition of the unwell pregnant woman + teamwork (observing and participating teams swap)	Drill	
12.45	Debrief (all teams)		
13.00	**Lunch**		
13.45	Obstetric haemorrhage + teamwork	Drill	
14.00	Major obstetric haemorrhage	Lecture	
14.30	Obstetric haemorrhage + teamwork (observing and participating teams swap)	Drill	
14.45	Debrief (all teams)		
15.00	**Tea/coffee break**		
	Teams move round to each of the four workshops as per timings on programme		

	Team 1	Team 2	Team 3	Team 4
15.15 – 15.35	Neonatal resuscitation	Shoulder dystocia	Vaginal breech/ twin birth	Fetal monitoring in labour
15.35 – 15.55	Shoulder dystocia	Vaginal breech/twin birth	Fetal monitoring in labour	Neonatal resuscitation
15.55 – 16.15	Vaginal breech/twin birth	Fetal monitoring in labour	Neonatal resuscitation	Shoulder dystocia
16.15 – 16.35	Fetal monitoring in labour	Neonatal resuscitation	Shoulder dystocia	Vaginal breech/ twin birth
16.35 – 16.45	General feedback Evaluation sheets Certificates			

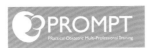

Example PROMPT course programme 2

Time	Programme	Format	Trainer/s
08.30	**Tea/coffee and registration**		
08.45	Introduction to course with team working Includes 'ice breaker'	Lecture	
09.15	Basic life support (all teams)	Instruction	
09.45	Severe hypertension/eclampsia scenario + teamwork	Drill	
10.00	Hypertensive disorders in pregnancy	Lecture	
10.30	Severe hypertension/eclampsia scenario + teamwork (observing and participating teams swap round)	Drill	
10.45	Debrief (all teams)		
11.00	**Tea/coffee break**		
11.15	Fetal monitoring in labour	Workshop	
11.45	Recognition of the unwell pregnant woman + teamwork	Drill	
12.00	Sepsis, recognition of the unwell pregnant woman	Lecture	
12.30	Recognition of the unwell pregnant woman + teamwork (observing and participating teams swap)	Drill	
12.45	Debrief (all teams)		
13.00	**Lunch**		
13.45	Obstetric haemorrhage + teamwork	Drill	
14.00	Major obstetric haemorrhage	Lecture	
14.30	Obstetric haemorrhage + teamwork (observing and participating teams swap)	Drill	
14.45	Debrief (all teams)		
15.00	**Tea/coffee break**		

Teams move round to each of the four workshops as per timings on programme

	Team 1	Team 2	Team 3	Team 4
15.15 – 15.35	Neonatal resuscitation	Shoulder dystocia	Cord prolapse	Maternal critical care
15.35 – 15.55	Shoulder dystocia	Cord prolapse	Maternal critical care	Neonatal resuscitation
15.55 – 16.15	Cord prolapse	Maternal critical care	Neonatal resuscitation	Shoulder dystocia
16.15 – 16.35	Maternal critical care	Neonatal resuscitation	Shoulder dystocia	Cord prolaspe
16.35 – 16.45	General feedback Evaluation sheets Certificates			

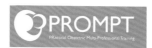

Example PROMPT course programme 3

Time	Programme	Format	Trainer/s
08.30	**Tea/coffee and registration**		
08.45	Introduction to course with team working Includes 'ice breaker'	Lecture	
09.30	Hypertensive disorders in pregnancy	Lecture	
10.00	Major obstetric haemorrhage	Lecture (APH or PPH)	
10.30	**Tea/coffee break**		
10.45	Maternal critical care and cardiac disorders	Lecture	
11.15	Sepsis, recognition of the unwell patient	Lecture and video	
11.45	Fetal monitoring in labour	Lecture and video	
12.30	**Lunch**		

Obstetric emergency workstations
30 minutes each station
Teams to follow workstation timetable for rotation to each station

	Team A	Team B	Team C	Team D	Team E	Team F
13.30 – 14.00	Obstetric haemorrhage + teamwork	Severe hypertension/ eclampsia + teamwork	Recognition of unwell pregnant woman + teamwork	Neonatal resuscitation	Shoulder dystocia (video + hands on)	Maternal critical care
14.00 – 14.30	Maternal critical care	Obstetric haemorrhage + teamwork	Severe hypertension/ eclampsia + teamwork	Recognition of unwell pregnant woman + teamwork	Neonatal resuscitation	Shoulder dystocia (video + hands on)
14.30 – 15.00	Shoulder dystocia (video + hands on)	Maternal critical care	Obstetric haemorrhage + teamwork	Severe hypertension/ eclampsia + teamwork	Recognition of unwell pregnant woman + teamwork	Neonatal resuscitation
15.00	**Tea/coffee break**					
15.15 – 15.45	Neonatal resuscitation	Shoulder dystocia (video + hands on)	Maternal critical care	Obstetric haemorrhage + teamwork	Severe hypertension/ eclampsia + teamwork	Recognition of unwell pregnant woman + teamwork
15.45 – 16.15	Recognition of unwell pregnant woman + teamwork	Neonatal resuscitation	Shoulder dystocia (video + hands on)	Maternal critical care	Obstetric haemorrhage + teamwork	Severe hypertension/ eclampsia + teamwork
16.15 – 16.45	Severe hypertension/ eclampsia + teamwork	Recognition of unwell pregnant woman + teamwork	Neonatal resuscitation	Shoulder dystocia (video + hands on)	Maternal critical care	Obstetric haemorrhage + teamwork
16.45 – 17.00	General feedback Evaluation sheets Certificates					

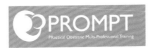

Example PROMPT course programme 4

Time	Programme	Format	Trainer/s
08.30	**Tea/coffee and registration**		
08.45	Introduction to course with team working Includes 'ice breaker'	Lecture	
09.30	Hypertensive disorders in pregnancy	Lecture	
10.00	Major obstetric haemorrhage	Lecture (APH or PPH)	
10.30	**Tea/coffee break**		
10.45	Maternal critical care work station	Practical session – case history in teams	
11.15	Sepsis, recognition of the unwell patient	Lecture and video	
11.45	Fetal monitoring in labour	Lecture and cases in teams	
12.30	**Lunch**		

Obstetric emergency workstations
30 minutes each station
Teams to follow workstation timetable for rotation to each station

	Team A	Team B	Team C	Team D	Team E	Team F
13.30 – 14.00	Obstetric haemorrhage + teamwork	Severe hypertension/ eclampsia + teamwork	Vaginal breech birth	Neonatal resuscitation	Shoulder dystocia (video + hands on)	Cord prolapse
14.00 – 14.30	Cord prolapse	Obstetric haemorrhage + teamwork	Severe hypertension/ eclampsia + teamwork	Vaginal breech birth	Neonatal resuscitation	Shoulder dystocia (video + hands on)
14.30 – 15.00	Shoulder dystocia (video + hands on)	Cord prolapse	Obstetric haemorrhage + teamwork	Severe hypertension/ eclampsia + teamwork	Vaginal breech birth	Neonatal resuscitation
15.00	**Tea/coffee break**					
15.15 – 15.45	Neonatal resuscitation	Shoulder dystocia (video + hands on)	Cord prolapse	Obstetric haemorrhage + teamwork	Severe hypertension/ eclampsia + teamwork	Vaginal breech birth
15.45 – 16.15	Vaginal breech birth	Neonatal resuscitation	Shoulder dystocia (video + hands on)	Cord prolapse	Obstetric haemorrhage + teamwork	Severe hypertension/ eclampsia + teamwork
16.15 – 16.45	Severe hypertension/ eclampsia + teamwork	Vaginal breech birth	Neonatal resuscitation	Shoulder dystocia (video + hands on)	Cord prolapse	Obstetric haemorrhage + teamwork
16.45 – 17.00	General feedback Evaluation sheets Certificates					

Appendix 2

Example PROMPT course certificate and evaluation sheet

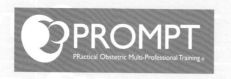

Local PROMPT Course

Date:
Venue:

This is to certify that.............................attended this training day

Subjects included:
Maternal Sepsis
Hypertensive disorders
Major obstetric haemorrhage
Shoulder Dystocia
Maternal Critical Care & cardiac disorders
Fetal Monitoring in Labour
Neonatal Resuscitation

Signed...(Local PROMPT Team)

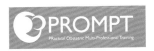

Local PROMPT course feedback sheet

Venue: ....

Date: ....

We would be grateful for your feedback on this PROMPT local course

Please tick one of the boxes for each question

Welcome and introduction with team working & ice breaker	Strongly agree	Agree	No opinion	Disagree	Strongly disagree
The introductory talk set the scene well					
The icebreaker activity was useful					
The content was about right					
Please briefly write one **'key' message** you have taken from this session:					
This session was useful					
The content was about right					
Please briefly write one **'key' message** you have taken from this session:					

Major obstetric haemorrhage	Strongly agree	Agree	No opinion	Disagree	Strongly disagree
The session was relevant to me					
The content was about right					
Please briefly write one **'key' message** you have taken from this session:					

Maternal critical care & cardiac disorders	Strongly agree	Agree	No opinion	Disagree	Strongly disagree
The session was relevant to me					
The content was about right					
Please briefly write one **'key' message** you have taken from this session:					

Sepsis & recognition of the unwell woman	Strongly agree	Agree	No opinion	Disagree	Strongly disagree
The session was relevant to me					
The content was about right					
Please briefly write one **'key' message** you have taken from this session:					

Fetal monitoring in labour	Strongly agree	Agree	No opinion	Disagree	Strongly disagree
The session was relevant to me					
The content was about right					
The example work station was useful					
Please briefly write one **'key' message** you have taken from this session:					

Shoulder dystocia practical workshop	Strongly agree	Agree	No opinion	Disagree	Strongly disagree
The session was relevant to me					
The content was about right					
The example work station was useful					
Please briefly write one 'key' message you have taken from this session:					

PPH drill & teamwork	Strongly agree	Agree	No opinion	Disagree	Strongly disagree
The session was relevant to me					
The content was about right					
The example work station was useful					
Please briefly write one 'key' message you have taken from this session:					

Recognition of the unwell woman drill & teamwork	Strongly agree	Agree	No opinion	Disagree	Strongly disagree
The session was relevant to me					
The content was about right					
The example work station was useful					
Please briefly write one 'key' message you have taken from this session:					

Maternal critical care work station	Strongly agree	Agree	No opinion	Disagree	Strongly disagree
The session was relevant to me					
The content was about right					
The example work station was useful					
Please briefly write one 'key' message you have taken from this session:					

Neonatal resuscitation	Strongly agree	Agree	No opinion	Disagree	Strongly disagree
The session was relevant to me					
The content was about right					
Please briefly write one 'key' message you have taken from this session:					

Severe hypertension/eclampsia & teamwork	Strongly agree	Agree	No opinion	Disagree	Strongly disagree
The session was relevant to me					
The content was about right					
Please briefly write one 'key' message you have taken from this session:					

Thank you for attending this local PROMPT course.

We value your feedback and welcome any ideas and/or comments about how the day could be improved.

Further feedback/comments

Appendix 3
Scenario props

Here are some examples and ideas for drill props for your scenarios.

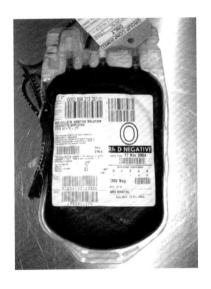

- **O-negative blood**

  Life-size laminated copy of a photo of an O-negative blood bag. You can loop through a treasury tag so that it can be hung from the drip stand, or alternatively put some Blu-Tack on the back.

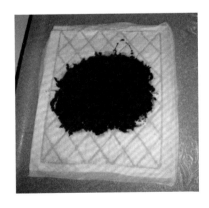

- **Bloodstained pads**

  Diluted red and blue food colouring can be poured onto incontinence pads and then dried. Once dry, they can be used repeatedly to simulate bloodstained sheets.

  Alternatively, green food colouring may be used to stain incontinence pads to look like offensive liquor for a sepsis scenario.

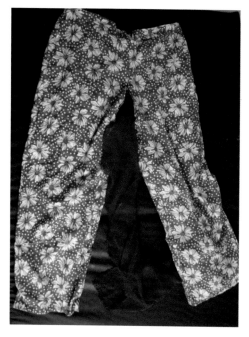

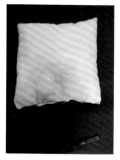 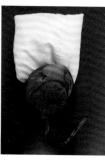

Magic cushion with 'uterus' inside
and then pulled out of cushion

- **Postpartum haemorrhage ('magic trousers')**

  Use two pairs of pyjama trousers, one pair inside the other, with the two waistbands attached to each other at four anchor points. Open the seam of the outside pair of trousers in the perineal area and feed a 3-metre strip of red lining material in between the two layers of one of the trouser legs. The bottoms of each of the trouser legs will also need sewing together so that the inner pair is attached to the outside pair, thus stopping the red lining material from falling out of the bottom of the trousers. The patient-actor wears the trousers and pulls out the red material periodically to signify haemorrhage.

- **Inverted uterus ('magic cushion')**

  You will need a large pink/red coloured bra (40DD) that has a separate cotton lining, and a small cushion.

  – Cut out the lining from each of the cups and shape into two circles. Sew these together to make the placenta (leave a small opening to enable some stuffing to be pushed inside the placenta).

  – Cut off one of the bra straps and attach this firmly to the placenta to make the cord.

  – Next open a 15 cm gap in the seam of the cushion. Take out a couple of handfuls of stuffing and use this to stuff the inside of the placenta. Sew up the placental opening. Use a blue marker pen to draw veins on the placenta and the cord.

  – Cut off all the straps and fastenings of the bra, so that you are left with just the two cups joined in the centre. Pin the two cups together so that they form a hollow heart-shaped uterus (shiny side of bra on

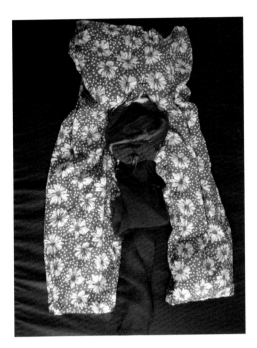

Magic cushion inside magic trousers, with inverted 'uterus' pulled out

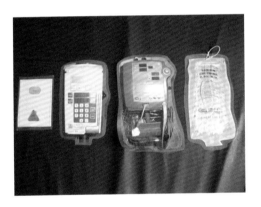

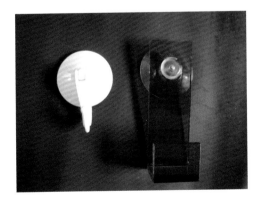

the outside) and then hand-sew them together. Once sewn together, firmly sew the placenta onto the top of the uterus.

– Finally, push the uterus inside out so that the placenta is now attached inside the uterus, and then push the whole uterus inside the opening of the cushion.

– Re-sew the cushion seam around the opening of the uterus so that it is firmly attached inside the cushion. The cushion can then be placed in between the two layers at the top of the magic PPH trousers and the cord and placenta can be pulled through the perineal opening, thus inverting the uterus.

- **Laminated photographs of local equipment**
  Here are examples of some of the laminated pictures of local equipment that can be attached to the wall (with Blu-Tack) if your labour rooms and/or key pieces of equipment aren't available for your drills. Any office or other clinical room can be used with the equipment pictures attached to walls and tables, so that staff will at least recognise their emergency call bell etc. These pictures are included in the *Items for printing*, but you may wish to take your own photos of your local equipment and laminate them.

- **Sticky hooks for hanging intravenous fluids and oxygen tubing etc.**
  If IV infusion stands aren't available for your drills, then suction hooks can be attached to the walls (shiny surfaces are best) and used for hanging IV fluids, oxygen masks and tubing and anything else that can be hung up.

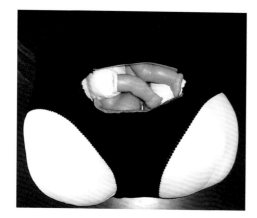

- **Perimortem caesarean section and cord prolapse ('magic pants')**

  Make a transverse cut in a large pair of maternity pants and line the cut with Velcro, so that the cut can be closed up again. The pants can be put on a mannequin and a baby doll and small cushion can be placed inside the pants to create a pregnancy. When a simulated perimortem caesarean section is necessary, the Velcro incision can be opened and the baby delivered.

  The magic pants may also be used in the cord prolapse scenario. The patient-actor can wear the magic pants over the magic trousers (with the red material pushed down the trouser leg so that it is not visible). The placenta from the PROMPT Flex, or even the magic cushion, can be placed inside the pants with a loop of cord hanging down to simulate the cord prolapse.

  If the baby from the magic pants is also used, then if the cord prolapse scenario proceeds to an urgent caesarean section, the birth of the baby can be simulated too.

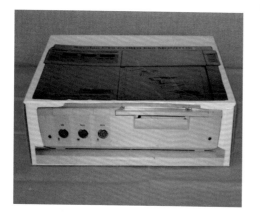

- **Cardboard-box CTG monitor**

  Take a photograph of the front and top of a CTG machine, print off the pictures (A4 size) and stick them on a cardboard box. Cover the box with sticky-backed plastic to make it more durable, or laminate the pictures before sticking them on the box. If available, real cardio- and toco-transducers can be attached to the patient-actor. The CTGs that have been provided in the downloadable materials for the relevant scenarios can be used with the box, or real CTG paper with a hand-drawn fetal heart rate recording can also be placed under the box and pulled out during the scenario, as required.

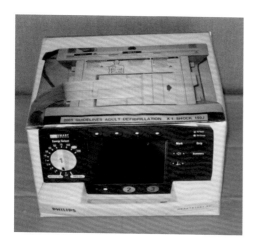

- **Cardboard-box defibrillator**

  As above, take photographs of the front and top of the defibrillator, stick the pictures onto the cardboard box and cover with sticky-backed plastic (or laminate the pictures first). Real defibrillator pads can be used with the fake machine so that the correct positioning of the pads on the mannequin can still be demonstrated and practised.

Index